Management in Rehabilitation

A Case-Study Approach

Management in Rehabilitation

A Case-Study Approach

Charles P. Schuch, MS, PT
Associate Professor Emeritus
Department of Physical Therapy
The University of North Carolina at Chapel Hill
Chapel Hill, North Carolina

Darlene K. Sekerak, PhD, PT
Clinical Associate Professor and Director
Department of Physical Therapy
The University of North Carolina at Chapel Hill
Chapel Hill, North Carolina

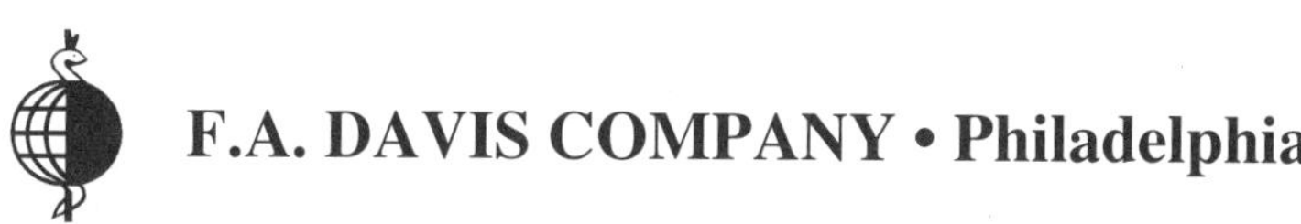

F.A. DAVIS COMPANY • Philadelphia

F.A. Davis Company
1915 Arch Street
Philadelphia, PA 19103

Printed in the United States of America

Last digit indicates print number: 10 9 8 7 6 5 4 3 2 1

Publisher, Allied Health: Jean-François Vilain
Developmental Editor: Crystal McNichol
Production Editor: Glenn L. Fechner
Cover Designer: Louis J. Forgione

Library of Congress Cataloging in Publication Data

Schuch, Charles P., 1928–
Management in rehabilitation : a case-study approach / Charles P. Schuch, Darlene K. Sekerak.
p. cm.
Includes index.
ISBN 0-8036-7758-8
1. Hospitals—Rehabilitation services—Personnel management—Case studies.
2. Rehabilitation centers—Personnel management—Case studies. 3. Management science—Case studies. I. Sekerak, Darlene K. II. Title.
RA975.5.R43S38 1996
362.1878680683—dc20 95-17209

My contribution to this book is dedicated to my wife, Hope, who has contributed so much to my life, and to our three fine sons, Doug, Jon, and Mike.

Charles P. Schuch

Foreword

Charles P. Schuch and Darlene K. Sekerak bring to this text a combination of knowledge and experience blended to create a concept-directed formula for problem resolution in PT and OT management situations. This text reflects the authors' concern for people, as well as their awareness and commitment to an orderly process in reaching effective outcomes. The 10-step problem-solving model recommended is not based entirely on empirical theory but is also grounded in the authors' years of experience using this approach. The information and strategies suggested are useful to the student as well as to the experienced PT or OT manager. I recommend *Rehabilitation in Management: A Case-Study Approach* to instructors as required reading and as a useful adjunct to traditional textbooks in administration.

In Part I, the authors employ a wide array of situations encountered by PT and OT managers on a regular basis as a means of facilitating the reader's awareness of, and involvement in, the decision-making process. The authors initially challenge the reader to consider the variety of factors impacting a given issue or situation and to creatively evaluate possible solutions using the 10-step problem-solving model. In Part II, the authors provide discussion about how they might approach the situation and offer concluding thoughts or "take home" lessons for the reader.

Chuck and Darlene are stalwart defenders of active learning and participatory management. This text is an excellent reflection of their teaching concepts, and it provides a realistic exposé of PT and OT management problems. I have appreciated the learning gained from my association with the authors and feel honored to write the Foreword for this text.

Robert C. Bartlett, PT, FAPTA
Professor and Chairman
Department of Physical and Occupational Therapy
Duke University
Durham, North Carolina

Preface

Problems are a regular occurrence in the management of people, no matter how expert the manager may be. The conviction that students and aspiring managers, if they are to be successful, must learn and practice a systematic approach to problem resolution provided the incentive for this text.

This book, which is a collection of case studies based in whole or part on true events, provides examples of problems of disharmony and friction. Problems born of opportunity, that is, problems resulting from of the existence of other problems are also presented.

Our primary goals in selecting cases for this book were:

1. To provide a model for the resolution of people problems in the health-care environment
2. To provide readers with the opportunity to practice their problem-solving skills and to study the issues associated with individual problems
3. To stimulate discussion among students about the methods of problem solving and the issues associated with individual problems

This is not a traditional textbook for a course in management. Rather, it is intended as a supplement to a traditional text. There is no one correct response to any of the cases. Within any group of individuals there will be differences in values, knowledge, and levels of confidence that may influence the analysis of information, the development and weighing of options, and decision making. The student should keep in mind that the process, rather than the choice of action, is of the essence.

We believe strongly that the values of the individuals involved in a problem should influence the different stages of the problem-solving process. We hope that the reader, through consideration of the problem situations presented in this book, will gain greater insight into his or her personal value system, as such an awareness is of great benefit when confronting actual situations of disharmony and friction.

Charles P. Schuch
Darlene K. Sekerak

Acknowledgments

The authors would like to thank the following reviewers for their helpful and suggestive comments: Kenneth D. Davis, PT, Assistant Administrator–Operations, Mid-America Rehabilitation Hospital, Overland Park, Kansas; Donna El-Din, PhD, PT, Professor, Department of Physical Therapy, Eastern Washington University, Cheney, Washington; Clyde B. Killian, PhD, PT, Director, Physical Therapy Program, Clarke College, Dubuque, Iowa; Frank McAdam Pierson, MA, PT, Emeritus, The Ohio State University, Columbus, Ohio; Ellen Berger Rainville, MS, OTR, FAOTA, Assistant Professor, Springfield College, Springfield, Massachusetts; and Janice E. Toms, Med, PT, Simmons College, Department of Physical Therapy, Boston, Massachusetts.

Also, special thanks to Jean-François Vilain, Allied Health publisher at F.A. Davis, and his staff for their support and encouragement.

Contents

CASE SCENARIOS

Steps 1–10

A Sample of the 10-Step Problem-Solving Process

During the past 50 years, researchers in management and administration have written volumes about problem solving. Much of this effort was in the industrial arena, very likely driven by the ever-increasing size of organizations, the complexity of doing business, and the tremendously high cost of failure to resolve problems in a timely and effective manner. Given the health-care industry's similar growth in size, complexity, and cost, much of the resultant information from research has applicability to the health-care environment.

What Is a Problem?

Despite the diversity of theories and approaches, a number of common themes emerge from the literature on problem solving. A problem exists when (1) the prevailing state is not what it should be or what one desires it to be and (2) when the cause or solution is not immediately known. Although widespread variance exists among authorities as to the best method of resolving a problem, there is reasonable consensus about the initial phases through which the problem solver must pass. These phases include (1) the recognition that a problem exists, (2) the recognition that one does not have an instant solution, and (3) the acknowledgment of a desire to resolve the problem.

In addition to being able to recognize the existence of a problem, the would-be solver, if he or she is to be effective, must be able to recognize and appreciate that there are different types of problems. The various categories into which problems may fall include:

Simple versus complex (i.e., determination of the need to add a single staff member versus determination of the need for departmental reorganization)

Quantifiable versus nonquantifiable (i.e., choosing between two computers versus choosing between two candidates for the position of Assistant Director)

Well-defined versus ill-defined (i.e., determination of adequacy of demand to justify a specified item of equipment versus dealing with what seems to be low morale)

Tame versus wicked* (determination of the color of mats to be purchased versus the matter of whether or not to go over your boss's head to appeal for additional space and personnel)

One point to be considered by the potential problem solver pertains to the matter of ownership. Not all problems belong in the lap of the highest authority. No manager should be expected to resolve every problem within his or her unit. The problem solver needs to determine early in the process "who owns the problem" and reassign the problem if necessary.

Problem Solving Versus Decision Making

An integral part of any problem-solving model is decision making. Decision making should not be perceived as being synonymous with problem solving. Decision making is the selection of an option from two or more options. Problem solving is the more comprehensive process by which the clinician or manager develops and analyzes alternatives before making a decision. Decision making, which may be considered the final stage in problem solving, is only one part of the problem-solving process.

The 10-Step Problem-Solving Process

Health-care providers have chosen people-oriented professions. Not surprisingly, many of the problems encountered by managers in health care are people-related; therefore they often tend to be complex, nonquantifiable, ill-defined, and all too often, wicked. A management problem can be approached most successfully in the same manner as a clinical problem, holistically rather than fragmentarily. The manager, like the clinician, must look beyond narrow and immediate implications and consider all the persons who might be involved. Students and novice managers would be wise to adopt a problem-solving model that makes it less likely that they will overlook any facets of the problem, which thereby enhances the prospect for successful resolution of the problem.

When entering the clinical phase of their education, students in the health-care professions learn early that a diagnosis does not necessarily define the patient's or

* A "wicked" problem has no definite description. There are many ways of defining the problem, and each one suggests a different direction in which to look for a solution. Every wicked problem can be thought of as a symptom of another problem. For additional information, see Rittell and Weber (1974). Cited by Hicks, MJ: Problem Solving in Business and Management. Chapman and Hall, New York, 1991.

client's problem. Labels such as multiple sclerosis, cerebrovascular accident, or even simple fracture fail to specifically identify the individual's complaints or limitations. Educators therefore present students with a systematic approach or model that serves as a guide in the evaluation of the individual's status, subsequent identification of problems, and the resolution of the problems identified. Analysis of problem-solving models suggests that although problem solving is a cognitive process, relying on rational and logical thought, it is (and should be) influenced significantly by experience, precedent, and values.

The 10-step linear problem-solving model that we recommend for use when confronted with management problems is shown in Figure 1. The literature describes numerous other models, but we chose this model as the most universally applicable and the most easily adopted by the novice manager.

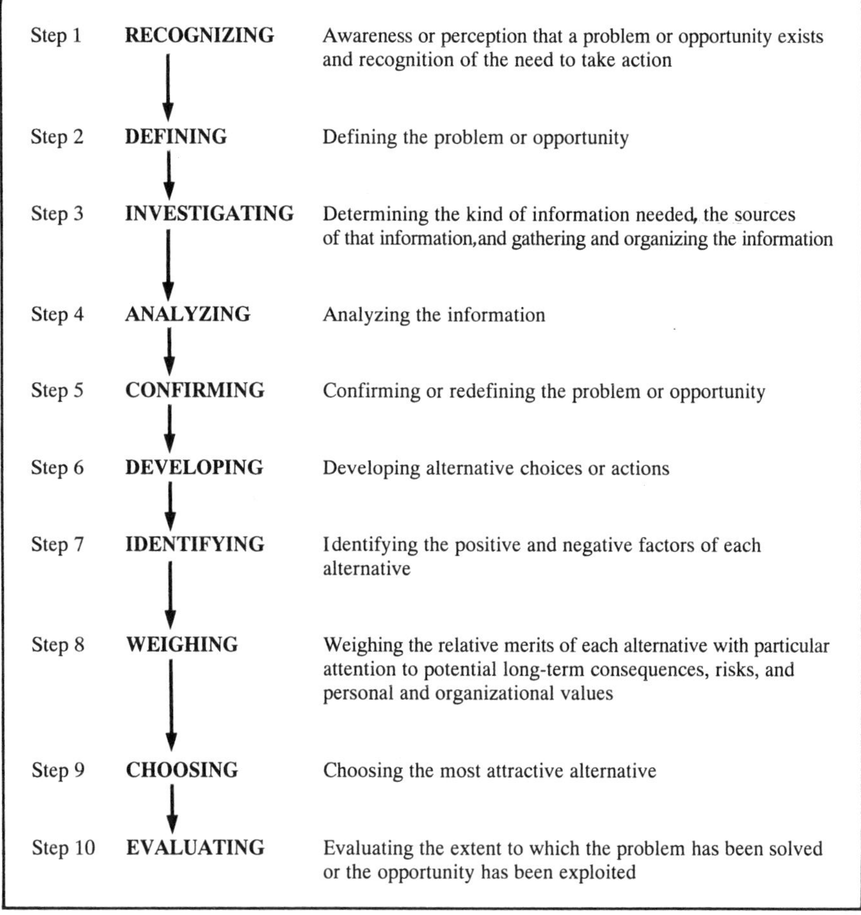

FIGURE 1

Each of the 10 steps listed is essential to effective problem solving. However, Steps 5 through 8 and Step 10 often receive insufficient attention from managers. For example, after gathering and analyzing information, the careful manager may determine that the originally perceived problem is not the true problem or that it represents only one facet of a complex situation. This manager recognizes the need to confirm or redefine the problem, but because of the time involved, does not develop a comprehensive slate of alternatives or carefully consider the positive and negative factors for each alternative. Our experience is that the investment of time and thought at Steps 5 through 8 can prevent many problems in the future. Ironically, many managers also overlook Step 10 and do not properly evaluate the extent to which the problem has been solved. This failure in follow-up can lead to regrettable repercussions if the problem later resurfaces. The time interval between decision making and evaluation is critical. It varies according to the problem and the reasonable time needed for the effects of the intervention to be evident. Many immediate resolutions are only temporary.

Some Important Considerations

The following five considerations are applicable to a problem-solving model in management:

1. Although a model may be based on rational and logical thought, it does not preclude the use of, or diminish the importance of, creative and intuitive thinking.
2. Managers would be wise to be mindful of their own individual values, including biases and prejudices, when proceeding through the problem-solving process. Personal biases may lead managers to confuse assumptions with facts or to misinterpret information critical to the problem-solving process.
3. Just as experienced clinicians often take shortcuts, combine several steps, and mentally rule out certain potential options, so do many experienced managers when grappling with an administrative problem. Experience, however, does not negate the need for a problem-solving model for either the experienced or inexperienced manager confronted with a complex, ill-defined, or nonquantifiable problem.
4. One often useful alternative that always merits consideration is to do nothing. Many perceived problems are resolved without intervention. In some circumstances, the interventions for perceived problems can create even larger, stickier problems. Weighing the consequences of inaction may also clarify the potential risks or benefits of alternative approaches.
5. Problems should not always be thought of in a negative light. They may be opportunities. For example, would you rather have a one-time gift of $1 million or 12 annual gifts of $100,000?

Are All Steps Necessary?

Experienced managers may rely on a condensed version with fewer steps. However, we caution students and young professionals with minimal management experience against the use of a condensed model. Greater specificity is more likely to encourage successful mastery of the problem-solving process, and each step is essential. The omission or neglect of any step may interfere with or prevent the successful resolution of a problem. Experienced managers may collapse the 10 steps into a more condensed model, but unless they attend to all components, they risk serious errors in judgment that may result in regrettable outcomes.

The Importance of Values

The cases presented in this book emphasize the type of "people problems" common to management in health care. Most managers, experienced and inexperienced alike, find people problems far more difficult to resolve than less personal issues such as budgets, space, and scheduling. People-related problems are complicated by a greater number of variables, foremost among them the interpersonal relationships and value systems of the parties involved. We would argue that the frequently heard reference to "personality conflict" often is a conflict of values rather than a conflict of respective personalities.

The value system of the organization and its management serves as a guide to the management style practiced and the priorities of the organizational unit. For example, the manager who values staff development is much more likely to be supportive of subordinates in continuing education and other career-enhancing opportunities. The manager who values his or her subordinates is much more likely to develop an effective two-way communication system and to respect input from subordinates.

Values relating to productivity and quality certainly influence patient scheduling and work performance evaluations. When the respective value systems of management and staff are compatible, the organizational environment is likely to be harmonious. In contrast, incompatible value systems are likely to result in disharmony and friction.

Organization of the Book

Part I provides a selection of cases describing realistic problems confronting health-care managers. The first and the last cases are presented in their entireties. All the pertinent information is presented in the sequential stages of the problem-solving process. The other cases are presented in various groupings according to the step(s) in the problem-solving process highlighted by the case. Instructors and students may prefer to select cases in a particular order based on their level of complexity or the topic under discussion. Readers are encouraged to respond, independently or in groups, to the questions and challenges presented in each case. The instructor should use the analyses and concluding thoughts in Part II to lead the students in a discussion of the case, making sure that all of the pertinent points, as featured in the analysis, are touched on. The students should not consult Part II until all individual or group effort has been exhausted.

SCENARIO: CASE 1

TRANSITIONS IN STYLE OF MANAGEMENT
Building Trust

Carla Smith, OT, was recently appointed director of a medium-sized occupational therapy department in a health maintenance organization (HMO). Upon accepting the position, Ms. Smith knew her predecessor had been unpopular with the staff and had been asked to resign because of staff discontent. With this information uppermost in Ms. Smith's mind, her highest priority was staff satisfaction. She wanted to manage the department in a way that allowed the staff to enjoy their work while providing a high level of service. As an advocate of participatory management, Ms. Smith decided to direct her initial efforts toward the staff's assessment of departmental status and suggestions for change.

At her first staff meeting Ms. Smith explained her preference for a participatory management style and expressed her sincere desire for input from all the members of the staff. She expressed the hope that everyone would contribute openly at staff meetings and in the individual conferences. She planned to schedule individual conferences with each member of the staff within the next 2 weeks. She then asked the staff to "get the ball rolling" by listing for her what they perceived to be the major strengths and weaknesses of the department. In particular, she asked them to identify the major problems confronting the department and to make suggestions to resolve those problems. Despite Ms. Smith's genuine efforts to elicit information from them, the staff was extremely noncommittal and offered nothing of substance. Ms. Smith closed the meeting by requesting that the staff think about objectives for the coming year, both individual and departmental. She suggested that they prepare to discuss individual goals with her in their respective one-on-one meetings.

During the ensuing 2 weeks Ms. Smith met with each staff member individually and conducted two staff meetings. To her great disappointment she observed a definite pattern of nonparticipation by all staff members. During this period staff were polite and reasonably pleasant to her and performed their duties acceptably. Nevertheless, they were reluctant to talk with her or to identify problems or objectives. No one challenged any of Ms. Smith's conclusions or suggestions, or intimated that they might have additional information that could be useful to her before she made a definite decision about an issue. Ms. Smith was particularly aware of a distinct air of uneasiness among staff members when they were in her office. Her greatest disappointment came from the failure of most of the staff to identify goals for the coming year, either individual or departmental.

Another 2 weeks passed with no significant change in staff behavior. Ms. Smith realized that the time was fast approaching when she would be required to submit departmental objectives and a proposed budget for the next fiscal year. The thought of that prospect caused Ms. Smith to conclude that she must deal with this problem. In an effort to resolve the perceived problem, Ms. Smith proceeded to work through a 10-step problem-solving process as follows:

Step 1—Recognizing

Is there a problem and must a decision be made? Ms. Smith believed there was a problem. More than a month had passed with no appreciable change in the extent of staff input to management. There was an approaching deadline for the submission of departmental objectives and proposed budget.

Step 2—Defining

"The staff does not contribute to a process of participatory management. How can I enlist their contributions to departmental objectives?"

Step 3—Investigating

Ms. Smith identified a number of persons within the hospital who she believed could offer helpful information and clues about why the staff members were so reluctant to participate. She met with the HMO administrator, the assistant administrator (Ms. Smith's immediate administrative superior), a number of physicians with close ties to the occupational therapy department, and a representative group of individuals from other departments with whom she had established rapport. The most salient items of information Ms. Smith gathered follow.

1. The staff harbored an intense dislike for the past director.
2. The past director was extremely autocratic in her management style and rarely permitted staff to participate in planning or decision making.
3. The past director was resentful of questions or unsolicited suggestions from the staff.
4. A vindictive climate existed in which the director found ways to punish those who disagreed with or challenged her ideas and actions.
5. The past director frequently belittled staff members for errors and new ideas.
6. Staff members were never invited into the director's office except for criticism or direct orders.

Step 4—Analyzing

Ms. Smith carefully reviewed the information provided by the persons interviewed. She was struck by the consistency of the information and by the clear pattern of behavior of her predecessor. At the conclusion of her review she believed she had a better understanding and appreciation for the following:

1. The lack of trust demonstrated by the staff
2. The absence of suggestions from the staff
3. The unease displayed by staff members in her office

Ms. Smith concluded that if she was to engage her staff in the management of their department, it was imperative that they develop an attitude of trust. She also concluded that the development of this trust would take time.

Step 5—Confirming

Given the conclusions drawn in Step 4, Ms. Smith redefined the original problem statement. "What can I do to get the staff to develop trust in me and contribute to the management of the department? What can I do to successfully solicit at least some staff input into departmental objectives?"

Step 6—Developing

Ms. Smith proposed the following alternatives.

Alternative 1

Take no specific action—simply wait for the passage of time to heal old wounds, calm old fears, and allow for the gradual development of rapport and trust.

Alternative 2

At the next departmental meeting make a frank statement of understanding of the department's past history and the reasons for the staff's lack of trust. In addition, explain her firm belief in a team concept and in participatory management. Follow this with an unequivocal pledge that she will not be guilty of the type of behavior exhibited by the former director.

Alternative 3

Develop a set of strategies, including the following:

a. Make a special effort in the next weeks and months to praise staff members publicly for positive performance, particularly for suggestions and constructive criticism.
b. Until greater rapport has been established, restrict constructive criticism of staff performance to a minimum.
c. On those occasions when constructive criticism of individuals is necessary, do it privately and with great tact.
d. Be highly tuned and receptive to comments and suggestions from staff members.
e. Be certain to implement at least some of any plans, goals, or suggestions emanating from the staff.
f. Deliver promptly on all promises made.
g. Praise the staff to higher administration in a manner that guarantees that the staff will learn of it.
h. Create a number of incentives to reward original ideas emanating from the staff.
i. Solicit staff input regarding objectives, plans, and changes through the use of multiple-choice ballots, rather than by use of open-ended or "either/or" formats.

These ballots should be completed anonymously, and collected and tallied by senior staff members before being relayed to the director. Questions might include:

1. I believe the number of referrals to the Out-Patient Hand Clinic can be increased in the next year by
   a. 5%
   b. 10%
   c. 15%
   d. ____
2. I believe the highest priority for the purchase of new equipment next year is
   a. An upper extremity isokinetic evaluation and exercise unit
   b. Personal computers and software
   c. Other ________________

Step 7—Identifying

Ms. Smith identified the following positive and negative factors associated with each alternative.

Alternative 1—Take No Specific Action

Positive Factors	*Negative Factors*
Pressure on the staff will be eased.	Possibility of staff input for the next fiscal year is minimized.
The staff develops trust and confidence at their own pace.	The staff may misinterpret Smith's backing off.
	Implementation of desirable changes or additions may be delayed.
	The director may make errors in judgment because of the lack of "insider" information withheld by the staff.

Alternative 2—Open Discussion With Staff

Positive Factors	*Negative Factors*
Development of more trust by some of the staff may result.	No significant negative repercussions are anticipated.
One or more of the less timid may begin to express ideas and be more forthcoming in the sharing of information	

Alternative 3a—Make Special Effort to Praise

Positive Factors	*Negative Factors*
Increased staff confidence is likely. Increased rapport between staff and Ms. Smith is a possibility. Increased trust by staff is a possibility.	No significant negative repercussions are anticipated.

Alternative 3b—Minimize Constructive Criticism of Staff

Positive Factors	*Negative Factors*
Staff tension is reduced.	The staff may misinterpret Ms. Smith's behavior and assume she is slack in her supervision or not very perceptive.
The prospect of staff learning to like Ms. Smith is enhanced.	There may be a delay in elevating the level of the quality of service and in implementing desirable changes.
A basis for trust may be established.	

Alternative 3c—Criticize Only Very Tactfully

Positive Factors	*Negative Factors*
Rapport is built.	No significant negative repercussions are anticipated.
Trust is developed.	

Alternative 3d—Be Receptive to Staff Comments and Suggestions

Positive Factors	*Negative Factors*
Staff confidence is increased.	No significant negative repercussions are anticipated.
Rapport is improved. Trust is developed by some or all staff. Basis for staff input is subtly increased.	

Alternative 3e—Implement Suggestions

Positive Factors	Negative Factors
Staff confidence is increased.	No significant negative repercussions are anticipated.
Rapport is improved.	
Trust is developed.	
Process of bonding for future staff participation in departmental management is begun.	

Alternative 3f—Prompt Fulfillment of Promises

Positive Factors	Negative Factors
Trust is developed.	No significant negative repercussions are anticipated.
Rapport is improved.	

Alternative 3g—Praise Staff to Higher Administration

Positive Factors	Negative Factors
Staff morale is improved.	No significant negative repercussions are anticipated.
Rapport is improved.	
Trust is increased.	

Alternative 3h—Reward Original Ideas

Positive Factors	Negative Factors
Sincerity regarding participatory management is demonstrated.	No significant negative repercussions are anticipated.
Trust is increased.	
Department benefits from new ideas.	

Alternative 3i—Utilize Multiple-Choice Responses

Positive Factors	Negative Factors
Anonymity reduces stress on staff.	Despite anonymity, making choices may be stressful to some.
Choosing from several choices as opposed to venturing an opinion is less stressful for staff.	Some may harbor resentment at being required to make choices.
Sincerity regarding staff input is demonstrated.	
Staff input contributes to plans for coming fiscal year.	
Trust is increased because of anonymity.	

Step 8—Weighing

The negative factors and risks associated with Alternative 1 concerned Ms. Smith. She concluded that this alternative offered too many opportunities for misunderstanding and misinterpretation of her motives. It also could unnecessarily delay resolution of the problem. Both Alternatives 2 and 3 were attractive. Ms. Smith anticipated no negative repercussions from Alternative 2 but expected a merely marginal positive outcome. Only the least timid and most adventurous risk takers among her staff were likely to respond. Her analysis of Alternative 3 suggested the possibility of negative factors associated with parts 3b and 3i, but overall, multiple opportunities for establishing a basis of trust and building rapport existed.

Step 9—Choosing

Ms. Smith chose Alternative 3 and began immediately to implement the strategies proposed. She solicited the assistance of the two most senior staff members to review and revise her multiple-choice questionnaire and to tally the responses.

Step 10—Evaluating

Ms. Smith recognized the need for dual approaches to evaluation. She kept records regarding her implementation of the strategies listed as part of Alternative 3 and of the response of the staff. Alternative 3 required multiple interventions, many requiring spontaneous responses by Ms. Smith to the staff. Ms. Smith realized her interpretation of the staff's response was dependent on her ability to evaluate the extent to which she had successfully implemented the strategies outlined. She kept a journal of her interactions with staff and noted the times she praised staff, responded to suggestions, and delivered on promises. She also recorded those times when providing constructive feedback or criticism was necessary. By referring to her journal, she was able to ensure that she did not omit anyone from those she praised and was able to keep track of staff concerns to be sure she responded promptly. She was particularly careful to incorporate the responses to the survey into the departmental goals and budget and to share both the survey responses and the proposed goals with the staff.

Ms. Smith recorded the number of times individual staff contributed to discussion or made suggestions in staff meetings and the number of unsolicited suggestions or amount of feedback she received from staff throughout the week. These records provided Ms. Smith with the information she needed to verify her gut reaction about the way the staff was responding to her intervention. Over the next several months a gradual but very clear trend was apparent. The staff, to Ms. Smith's delight, was clearly becoming more involved in the management of the department. She looked forward to a more enthusiastic response when the opportunity to plan annual goals arrived next year.

Steps 1–2

Recognizing and Defining a Problem

SCENARIO: CASE 2

REGULAR STAFF VERSUS CONTRACT PERSONNEL
Coping With Conflict

City Memorial Hospital is a 400-bed acute-care hospital located in the older and poorer section of Gothem, an area with the highest crime rate in the city. Once the jewel in the city's hospital system, City Memorial now resembles the environment in which it is located. It appears old and past its prime. The rehabilitation department, although well-endowed with space and equipment, reflects the hospital and its external environment. It is a gloomy, cheerless-looking place.

For the past several years, the rehabilitation department has been budgeted for ten physical therapists, seven occupational therapists, three speech pathologists, and for assistants and other support staff. Because of the less-than-cheerful internal and external environment and the intense competition for rehabilitation professionals, the department was consistently short-staffed by four to six positions. This 20 to 30 percent shortage of therapists has taken its toll over time, resulting in tension from overloaded schedules, frequent overtime, and shortened lunch breaks. The major consequences include an excessive turnover rate among the professional staff, increased absenteeism, a decline in the frequency and quality of patient documentation, and a stagnating performance improvement program.

At one of the less and less frequently held staff meetings 6 months ago, a lively discussion took place. The professional staff unanimously expressed their discontent with the existing conditions and demanded that the shortage of personnel be resolved.

Six physical therapists and two occupational therapists threatened to resign if things did not change within the next 3 months.

Marge Pullen, director of rehabilitation, has been at City Memorial for 12 years and has been head of the department for the past 5 years. Despite the continuing shortage of staff, she is considered a good manager by hospital officials and the department staff. She, too, felt the effects of the shortage of personnel and was aware that her administrative activities and effectiveness suffered because she significantly increased the percentage of her time involved in direct patient care activity at the expense of administration. She also realized she was rapidly becoming "burned out." Consequently, she was neither surprised nor angry at the demands of the staff and, though regretful, she was understanding of the threats of resignation. She was fully aware that something had to be done.

The first thing Ms. Pullen did was to consider the matter of recruitment of additional therapists. She thoroughly reviewed and was satisfied that her department's salary scale and fringe benefits compared favorably with the competing services in the area, with the exception of the organizations that provided contract services. She reviewed her recruitment efforts and concluded that little could be done to improve these efforts. Although there were numerous responses to local and national advertisements, many of the prospects declined offers because they were unimpressed by the appearance of the department and concerned about the high crime rate in the neighborhood. She decided that, difficult as it might be to physically change an old structure, an effort must be made to make the department look more cheerful for employees and patients. Faced with the serious decline of staff morale and the credible threat of resignation from almost half of her therapists, Ms. Pullen also concluded that she must take steps to quickly alleviate the staff shortage. She made an appointment to discuss her problem with Mr. Carson, the administrator of the hospital.

When Ms. Pullen met with Mr. Carson she painstakingly reviewed the plight of her department and tried to impress him with the need to make physical changes in the department to improve esthetics and, of even greater urgency, to take action immediately to hire more therapists and forestall a major disaster. She presented Mr. Carson with suggestions concerning the physical renovation of the department and a formal proposal from a contract organization for the provision of three full-time-equivalent (FTE) physical therapists and one and a half FTE occupational therapists. The cost to the department was equal to the amount currently budgeted for the six positions now vacant. The proposal was the best of several solicited by Ms. Pullen, and it provided strong assurance of supplying the 4.5 FTEs within 2 weeks after signing the contract. Although regretting that the 4.5 FTEs were less than the budgeted and needed 6.0 FTEs, Ms. Pullen recommended acceptance of the proposal as an alternative far superior to maintaining the status quo. Mr. Carson was readily convinced of the merit of the recommendation and told Ms. Pullen to proceed with the contract. He also agreed to her suggestions for improving the appearance of the department.

Ms. Pullen, given the green light by Mr. Carson, completed the negotiations with Therapy Providers, Inc. (TPI) and within the prescribed 2 weeks TPI provided two full-time and two part-time physical therapists and two part-time occupational therapists to meet its commitment. The immediate reaction of the regular departmental staff was one of delight. After the first week of orientation and settling in by the contract therapists, the "regulars" were pleased and relieved to have more time for patient care and documentation. The staff experienced a reduction in overtime and stress.

Things went along well for a brief period, and although the contract personnel irked the regulars in a number of ways, the regulars were forgiving because of the tangible and intangible benefits from the contract. As the months passed, however, the complaints escalated and ended the "honeymoon." Departmental regulars elected a delegation of three to address their complaints to Ms. Pullen. The list of complaints presented to Ms. Pullen was lengthy and diverse.

1. **Department policies and procedures.** Contract personnel, either through ignorance or by design, often violated policies and procedures. It was particularly irksome to the regulars to see these violations ignored or forgiven by the director.
2. **Treatment regimens.** Contract personnel often employed treatment regimens different from the regulars. The regulars implied they could accept these differences in most cases, but not when they were out of compliance with a treatment regimen initiated by a regular.
3. **Rigid adherence to the clock.** The regulars complained that contract personnel always left the department at precisely 5 PM, never staying late for overloads or late referrals. The contract therapists explained their behavior by referring to the terms of the contract that called for a specific number of hours of service. As a result, the regulars frequently had to work past 5 PM.
4. **Assisting regular staff.** The regulars resented the tendency of contract personnel to fail to volunteer to help regulars when the latter were pressed for time.
5. **Overload.** The regulars alleged that the contract therapists resisted assuming a schedule overload on those occasions when regulars were absent for any reason.
6. **Criticism of regulars' skills.** Some of the contract therapists were overheard making derogatory remarks about the knowledge and level of performance of some of the regulars.
7. **Staff meetings.** Two of the contract therapists did not attend staff meetings (not scheduled on their work days) and this created problems when they were unaware of items discussed at the meeting. It was also alleged that the contract therapists in attendance were inattentive and rarely participated in discussions.
8. **Caseload.** The regulars were unanimous in citing specific examples of contract personnel avoiding certain patients or types of conditions.
9. **Social interaction.** The regulars complained about the contract therapists "hanging around together" and failing to join in social activities of the department.
10. **Salary discrepancy.** The regulars harbored resentment that the contract therapists were paid at a higher rate and enjoyed a more liberal benefits package.

After the presentation and explanation of the complaints, the delegates proceeded to present their demands as follows:

1. Contract personnel must adhere to all policies and procedures and to workload and overtime expectations.
2. The salary schedule for the hospital-employed therapists must be adjusted to the level of the contract therapists.

Ms. Pullen listened to the delegates and indicated she could not make an immediate response to the demands. She did promise to review the complaints carefully, consider the demands, and respond within 5 to 10 workdays. The delegation accepted this plan and thanked Ms. Pullen for her time and concern.

Later in the day when her schedule offered the opportunity for meditation in the privacy of her office, Ms. Pullen began to reflect on the meeting with the staff representatives. She experienced a dejected sense of being between the proverbial rock and a hard place. Because of shortages, staff came to her with a demand for an immediate relief of the stressful conditions. She responded by entering into a contractual arrangement that alleviated the personnel shortage. But now, after only a few months, the staff is once again discontent and has presented a new set of demands. After a period of wandering thoughts, including an awareness of a 10 percent salary discrepancy between the two groups of therapists, Ms. Pullen pulled her thoughts together and acknowledged to herself, "I know I have to do something." Having recognized the presence of a problem and the need to make one or more decisions, she is ready to progress to Step 2—defining the problem.

How would you define the problem?

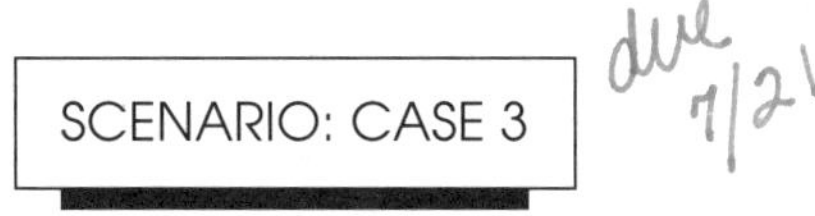

WHAT WENT WRONG?
Delegation

Phil Bassett, MS, PT, was the proud owner of Bassett Physical Therapy Service in a large metropolitan area. After receiving his physical therapy license, he worked for several years in a large hospital, first as a staff therapist and later as a team leader. He then became the director of physical therapy at a smaller hospital with a department of ten employees, including seven physical therapists. After 2 years he wanted to be his own boss and have more involvement with athletic injuries. He studied his community's demographics and spoke with a number of local physicians and healthcare payor organizations about the possibility of opening a private practice. He listened carefully to the suggestions of the orthopedists who treated many of the athletic injuries in the community. Mr. Bassett decided to take a chance. He opened a private practice in a medical office complex that housed a large number of orthopedists and other medical practitioners.

Mr. Bassett's move was a good one. The combination of his convenient location, a good relationship with the key orthopedic physicians, and his interest and expertise in athletic injuries resulted in the immediate use of his services and rapid growth.

Over the next 3 years he demonstrated his entrepreneurship by working with other physicians and provider networks in the community to develop a number of specialized programs not offered elsewhere in the community. To implement and maintain those specialized programs, he recruited effectively and employed a cadre of highly skilled physical therapists. As the specialized programs and the practice grew, Mr. Bassett's complement of physical therapists grew to ten. What had been an operation with one physical therapist 3 years ago was now an organizational entity of ten physical therapists, two physical therapist assistants, and various clerical personnel.

By the end of the third year, Bassett Physical Therapy Service was a huge financial and clinical success, but not all was bliss! Phil Bassett began his enterprise as a very simple organization with only a receptionist. Although the practice grew and he continued to add personnel, the basic organizational structure remained the same. He was the boss, and all employees were responsible directly to him. This approach worked efficiently for a time, but with continued expansion Mr. Bassett spent more time in his office and less time in the treatment area. As a result, he was less accessible to his staff. This led to a number of problems. Furthermore, in recruiting to meet the personnel needs of specialized programs, Mr. Bassett was not consistent in his hiring practices, nor in his allocation of salary increments and bonuses. These inconsistencies led to friction among some of the staff. A number of other operational problems also arose relating to scheduling, use of equipment, work hours, and leave time.

Mr. Bassett recognized the increasing unrest among his employees and was genuinely concerned. A mass exodus of staff would be very detrimental to the practice. After pondering the matter, he belatedly came to the conclusion that his practice had grown beyond the scope of its original organization. He could no longer be solely responsible for the entire operation or the only person to whom all others answered. Faced with this conclusion, Mr. Bassett decided to take action.

The first step taken by Mr. Bassett was to appoint Ann Gray, PT, Director of Clinical Operations and to put her in charge of the daily operations of the clinic. In addition to coordinating the daily operation of the clinic, Ms. Gray was charged with specific responsibility for supervising all physical therapy personnel and developing work performance standards, evaluation documents, and a performance improvement program. Mr. Bassett informed her that in addition to other responsibilities of ownership and management, he would develop a table of organization and a policy and procedure manual.

Mr. Bassett selected Ms. Gray for promotion for reasons that he considered to be apparent and logical. Ms. Gray was on his staff at the hospital before he opened his private practice, and she was the first addition to his expanding practice. He knew her to be a conscientious professional, with advanced knowledge and skill. Ms. Gray had a pleasant demeanor and always got along well with her colleagues and Mr. Bassett. Although she had no prior administrative experience, Mr. Bassett was confident that Ms. Gray's intelligence, tact, reputation, and work ethic more than qualified her for the newly created position.

A period of 6 months passed during which the practice continued to thrive. Mr. Bassett completed the table of organization and the policy and procedure manual. The completion of those tasks coincided with the approaching end of the fiscal year. He decided this was the ideal time to meet with Ms. Gray to see what she had developed and to implement the work performance evaluation (WPE) process as a basis for determining salary increments for the coming fiscal year. He eagerly set a date for the two of them to meet.

The day of the meeting arrived, and Mr. Bassett entered the conference room with great enthusiasm. He greeted Ms. Gray cheerfully and with no further ado said, "OK, show me what you have." Ms. Gray hesitated and then blurted out that she had not yet completed any of the projects delegated to her. After a moment of stunned silence Mr. Bassett blew his stack and berated Ms. Gray for letting him down and failing to live up to her responsibilities. He demanded an explanation. Ms. Gray responded that she was so busy with the operation of the clinic that she was unable to concentrate on the special projects. Her patients and the running of the clinic occupied so much of her time that the staff was complaining about her inaccessibility. When forced to choose in scheduling her time, Ms. Gray admitted that she always gave priority to her patients, believing she could catch up on the administrative tasks. Not only did Mr. Bassett's bubble of enthusiasm burst on hearing this, but he felt that he and his practice were worse off now than they were 6 months ago. What went wrong?

Define the problem. Identify and discuss the errors of omission and commission that contributed to this calamity at Bassett Physical Therapy Service.

SCENARIO: CASE 4

DECLINING WORK PERFORMANCE
Concern for the Individual

Roberta Gonzalas, PT, as director of rehabilitation services at Central Hospital, is responsible for the management of a physical and occupational therapy department employing 70 persons. There is a secretarial staff of six, including Ms. Jane Parsons, whose official title is administrative assistant. Ms. Parsons, a 61-year-old widow who first joined the department as a secretary 22 years ago, has served in her present capacity for the past 15 years. She is loyal, efficient, and self-motivated, and she provides excellent supervision of other support staff. She is popular among all departmental personnel and a great ambassador for the department throughout the hospital. Ms. Gonzalas regards Ms. Parsons as an outstanding person and administrative assistant.

About 2 years ago, a number of subtle changes in Ms. Parson's behavior began to occur. She now frequently arrives late for work. Support staff, much to their surprise and dismay, note uncharacteristic episodes of impatience. Ms. Gonzalas observes that Ms. Parsons is not always as efficient as in the past; she seems to be having difficulty adapting to the rapid expansion of the department and the many recent changes incorporated by Ms. Gonzalas and the hospital administration.

Since the onset of these behavioral irregularities, Ms. Parsons' work performance has steadily declined. This was dutifully, though regretfully, recorded in her last two work performance evaluations (WPEs). The most recent recording was about a week ago.

During the WPE conference, Ms. Gonzalas reviewed the specific items and the ratings. She said, "Jane, I am concerned about you, not simply as an employer, but also as a friend. I know there must be a reason for the decline in your work performance and in your relationships with your associates. I want to help you, but I can't unless you tell me what is at the root of these changes. Please tell me."

Ms. Parsons deliberated for a moment and then, accepting the sincerity of Ms. Gonzalas's plea, decided to level with her. The gist of Ms. Parson's response follows:

> I know that I am not as good an administrative assistant as I once was. But then, the job and the work environment are not the same. Nor am I the same person physically or mentally. My physical condition has deteriorated because of aging to a certain extent, but primarily because of arthritis. There are many mornings when it takes all my will power to get out of bed and get moving. I don't move as fast as I used to. There are days when I physically ache to the point of distraction.
>
> I used to love this job and always looked forward to coming to work. It was my salvation after my husband died. But that's not true anymore. Now I almost dread coming to work! This place has become such a bureaucratic nightmare that the simplest task or request results in a blizzard of paper. All the new rules, regulations, and paperwork passed on by administration, the Feds, and third-party payers, as well as constant changes in procedures, doubles and triples the volume of work to be done. We have become totally computer dependent, and I am so busy I don't have time to learn all the nuances of computer operations. Being a product of the old typewriter age, I am scared to death of the computer. I can just feel my stress level rising when I have to grapple with the monster.
>
> Another frustration relates to my staff. There was a time when there was very little turnover. I knew that when I oriented and trained a person he or she would be around long enough to produce good work and be a real help to me. But now the younger folks take a job with us to get experience as a stepping stone to something better. The constant turnover occupies more and more of my time in training.
>
> Because the department has grown so much, there is much more work to be done, and though we have added clerical staff it has not been in proportion to the growth of professional staff. For example, 5 years ago we

> had clinical affiliations with 8 physical therapy schools and 5 occupational therapy schools. Now we have affiliations with 26 physical therapy schools and 18 occupational therapy schools. That makes triple the work for me in handling the administrative aspects of clinical education. I don't feel I can delegate any of that work because the rest of the staff is overwhelmed as well.
>
> With the size and turnover rate of staff, the work environment is far less personal and friendly than it used to be. Frankly, I feel under great stress, which doesn't help my arthritis a bit, and I seriously question my ability, physically, mentally, and emotionally, to perform this job at the level you and I believe appropriate.

Ms. Gonzalas was disturbed at hearing this lengthy recitation by Ms. Parsons. She was concerned about the position of administrative assistant and the efficient discharge of the responsibilities associated with it, but she was even more concerned about Ms. Parsons and her physical and mental health. During the ensuing discussion, Ms. Gonzalas learned or verified a number of relevant factors.

1. Ms. Parsons' arthritis was not of such a debilitating state as to qualify her for disability retirement.
2. Ms. Parsons did not feel she could retire at this time because:
   a. She would not be eligible for social security for another year.
   b. If she were to retire at age 62, her monthly social security benefits would be reduced by 19 percent.
   c. She is not eligible by age or years of service for retirement benefits from the hospital.
   d. Mr. Parsons' estate was insufficient to provide a decent living standard without full social security benefits and the hospital's retirement plan.
   e. Ms. Parsons did not have many outside interests and feared she would not be happy in retirement at this time, even if she could afford it.

Ms. Gonzalas thanked Ms. Parsons for her frankness and her willingness to discuss her situation. She pledged to weigh the matter and get back to her soon. Ms. Gonzalas is fully aware that she has a problem.

How would you define Ms. Gonzalas' problem?

SCENARIO: CASE 5

ROMANCE IN THE WORKPLACE
Who Owns This Problem?

Walkertown Clinic is a large outpatient physical and occupational therapy practice in the sprawling suburb of Walkertown. It was started by owners Peter Jordan,

MS, PT, and Cindy Crowly, MA, OT/R, 20 years ago. The original business has grown into a profitable small corporation, Southwest Orthopedic. The corporation now has 42 satellites in small cities and towns across the Southwest and West. Walkertown Clinic employs 12 physical therapists (PTs), 2 physical therapist assistants (PTAs), 7 occupational therapists (OTs), 3 certified occupational therapy assistants (COTAs), a business manager, and 3 office personnel. Stephanie Reona, PT, is the clinical director of Walkertown Clinic and five of the more geographically proximate satellites. Southwest Orthopedic corporate offices, and consequently Mr. Jordan's and Ms. Crowly's offices, are located in the same building as the Walkertown Clinic.

Ms. Reona accepted the position of clinical director with Walkertown 7 years ago. She was attracted by the clinic's dynamic and energetic staff, the owners' support of the professional advancement of the staff, the encouragement and inducements for clinical research, and the absolute commitment to value in services for patients. The quality of care at Walkertown impressed Ms. Reona as the best she had seen anywhere. Seven years later she is still pleased about her choice and grateful for the opportunity to have served in a leadership role in an exciting and challenging health-care corporation.

Both Mr. Jordan and Ms. Crowly are outstanding mentors and role models. They outline the general goals, standards for quality, and guiding principles for operation. They encourage the hiring of professionals who share their values, and then express their confidence in those individuals by allowing them to work independently to meet the company's goals. They are lavish with their recognition for accomplishment and responsive to the expressed concerns of employees.

Mr. Jordan and Ms. Crowly live relatively conservative personal lives. The business requires considerable travel, but they share the burden equally. They both prefer quiet weekends at home with their families. Mr. Jordan has been married for 18 years and has four children, the oldest of which will be starting college next fall. Ms. Crowly was married 3 years ago to an attorney in town, and the two still appear to be enjoying an extended honeymoon.

Ms. Reona and her husband are close personal friends with the Jordans and the Crowlys. They often are guests at each others homes and have vacationed together at the coast for several years. These relationships further reinforce Ms. Reona's satisfaction with her job and her overall association with Walkertown.

A month ago, Mr. Jordan made a most unusual request of Ms. Reona. One evening when both were working late, Mr. Jordan dropped by Ms. Reona's office for causal conversation on his way to the kitchen area for a cup of coffee. This was by no means unusual. On this particular evening, however, he asked Ms. Reona for a favor, the kind of favor he had never requested in the past. The Walkertown Clinic had a vacancy for a COTA. Mr. Jordan asked Ms. Reona to transfer Sally Winthrop, COTA, from a smaller satellite clinic across town and fill the vacant position at the satellite with a new employee. Mr. Jordan did not justify his request, but simply asked Ms. Reona to look into the matter and give it some consideration. The next day Ms. Reona found a letter on her desk from Ms. Winthrop requesting a transfer to the main clinic because of its proximity to her home.

Ms. Reona knew Ms. Winthrop and recalled that her work performance evaluations were always excellent. She related well to the staff and was exceptional with patients in both rapport and clinical skills. She found no reason not to grant Ms. Winthrop's request and arranged for her transfer.

Ms. Winthrop was well-received by the Walkertown staff and fit in immediately. Patients and therapists raved about her. She was conscientious about her documentation and often stayed late to tidy up in anticipation of the next day's schedule of patients. On a number of occasions Ms. Winthrop was still there rinsing out cups or reviewing her notes when Ms. Reona left for the day.

During the past 2 weeks the chatter in the business office increased, and there were obvious whisperings going on at the therapists' workstation. Ms Reona assumed it had something to do with a surprise party being planned for one of the occupational therapists who was leaving at the end of the week. Over a cup of coffee with one of the staff therapists, Ms. Reona asked what all the whispering was about. The therapist's response was "Don't you know? Mr. Jordan is having an affair with Sally Winthrop! Everyone is talking about it."

Ms. Reona collected her purse, signed out for the afternoon, and went to the park to think.

Define the problem. Whose problem is it?

SCENARIO: CASE 6

THE JOKE'S ON YOU
Harassment in the Workplace

Doug Rosetti is supervisor of speech language and audiology in the Snow County Public School System. The system serves 42 local schools and employs 30 speech/language pathologists and three audiologists. Mr. Rosetti has been with the System for 13 years. He is well liked by the administration, recognized for his insistence on quality services for children, and respected among his professional peers for his success in acquiring local salary supplements for his therapists. Turnover among therapists at Snow County is typical for most school systems, and many of the therapists there have less than 2 years experience. Recruitment of new therapists is rarely difficult. This is attributed to Mr. Rosetti's reputation as a fair and respected leader, competitive salaries, and a supportive professional work environment.

Mr. Rosetti works many long hours at the office, developing proposals for new programs, consulting with therapists about service delivery problems, and tracking staff productivity, looking for ways to optimize services to children. In spite of his seriousness and commitment about his work, Mr. Rosetti maintains a casual office demeanor and attempts to keep the atmosphere in the office relaxed and easygoing. He tries to reduce the stress of heavy caseloads and tricky interdisciplinary relationships in the schools with an office oasis that is comfortable and informal. He encourages celebrations for even minor accomplishments by staff and publicly acknowledges effort as well as success. Many of these acknowledgments are packaged in the form of a gag gift or humorous certificate of merit or appreciation.

Mr. Rosetti is perceived to be a warmhearted man who takes a sincere interest in everyone. He is never too busy to make time to listen to a therapist with a concern. He always listens attentively. He shows his compassion and interest with eye contact and often with a reassuring stroke or pat on the shoulder. He acknowledges the employee's feelings and always offers some suggestion to move toward a solution. He is the first to recognize if someone is feeling low or if a therapist is sporting a new haircut or an engagement ring. The staff seems to appreciate his personal interest. When he returns from state professional association meetings, they are always eager to hear his latest repertoire of new and somewhat-off-color jokes and humorous stories. When a staff person has been out of the office for an extended vacation or illness, it is not uncommon for Mr. Rosetti to welcome the person back with a warm, fatherly hug.

Myra Hopkins is a speech and language pathologist hired 3 months ago to fill a new position added as a result of the increasing number of students in the elementary schools in the northern portion of the county. Ms. Hopkins moved to Snow County from the Midwest, where she worked in a much smaller school district for her first 2 years following graduation. Her letters of recommendation described her as quiet but personable and noted her exceptional clinical skills, especially in the area of oral motor and feeding programs for severely multihandicapped children. She also had some experience with assistive technology and computer-learning applications for children with disabilities. These specialized skills made her most attractive for employment.

Ms. Hopkins seems to be adjusting to Snow County with ease. Joan Rankowski, the therapist responsible for Ms. Hopkins orientation, shared very favorable comments from principles, teachers, and students. Ms. Rankowski was particularly impressed with the manner in which Ms. Hopkins handled her first Individual Educational Plan (IEP) meeting with a child's parents and the other interdisciplinary team members. The parents were particularly emotional about a recommendation for a new placement. Ms. Hopkins was effective in allaying their fears and in helping them to focus on the goals for the child and the advantages of the recommended placement for meeting those goals.

Mr. Rosetti noted that Ms. Hopkins was still very reserved around the office and particularly around him. He recalled the comments from her recommendation letters about her quiet personality and concurred with the previous employer's assessment. Her personality certainly did not seem to have any adverse effects on her work. Mr. Rosetti made an effort to be friendly and to compliment Ms. Hopkins on her appearance and her work, as he did all other therapists in the office. He made an extra effort to include her in office conversations or outings for lunch.

When Ms. Hopkins first arrived in Snow County she took advantage of her "new life" to tackle a stubborn problem she had with her weight. She signed up for support from a local diet clinic and is pleased at her success. Over the past 3 months she has lost 30 of her targeted 37 pounds. The change in her appearance is quite dramatic.

Late Friday afternoon the staff gathered for a weekly staff meeting and, as was customary, Mr. Rosetti gave out the awards for the week. He included among them an award for the sexiest new figure and presented it to Ms. Hopkins. She glared at him and left without taking the certificate or saying good-bye. The group seemed puzzled and offended by her response. Mr. Rosetti was worried.

As he feared, Ms. Hopkins was waiting for him when he arrived at work on Monday morning. She informed him that she considered his tasteless humor and cheap advances as sexual harassment. She intended to file a formal complaint with the system's Personnel Office that morning. She walked out of his office before he had a chance to respond. Mr. Rosetti immediately remembered a poster he had seen at the last supervisors' meeting. It read, SEXUAL HARASSMENT—EVERY MANAGER'S NIGHTMARE."

Is there a problem? How would you define it?

SCENARIO: CASE 7

WHAT ARE YOU GOING TO DO ABOUT IT?
Respect for Delegated Authority

Metropolitan Medical Center includes a 700-bed multifaceted hospital, a trauma center, a subacute facility, and multiple specialized outpatient services. It is located in a large southern city. The medical center has an outstanding reputation among its clientele and peer organizations, attributed to the excellence of care offered and the diversity and comprehensiveness of diagnostic and treatment programs. Though in existence for nearly a century, the center occupies a complex of relatively new and well-designed buildings, with easy access to the community and with generous parking space.

Consistent with the overall quality and diversity of the center, the Department of Rehabilitation also enjoys an excellent reputation among patients, peers, and physicians. This large department, in addition to providing general acute care, includes specialized programs in physical rehabilitation, cardiac rehabilitation, pediatrics, neurology, back pain, athletic injuries, cardiopulmonary intensive care, and trauma. Little wonder that the Department of Rehabilitation of Metropolitan Medical Center is a highly desirable setting for the clinical education of occupational therapy and physical therapy and speech/language and audiology students. In fact, the department has formal affiliations with 20 schools, and it has turned down many others in an effort to keep the clinical education program manageable and of high quality.

The well-organized and active clinical education program at Metropolitan accepts students at various stages of their education program—early, mid, and late. The department provides interdisciplinary clinical education learning experiences in each of its specialty services. The clinical education program is under the direction of Linda Branch, OT/R, the center coordinator for clinical education (CCCE). Ms. Branch coordinates all requests from schools for clinical education and fieldwork assignments and frequently pairs teams of occupational and physical therapy students with clinical instructors (CIs) based on a set of guidelines mutually agreed on by the director of rehabilitation, the faculty coordinators at affiliating schools, team leaders, and CIs. The prevailing opinion is that Ms. Branch is organized, efficient, effective, and fair.

Several months ago the lead therapist in the Trauma Center resigned. The Trauma Center is an 18-bed unit that handles severe acute trauma cases, including spinal cord injuries, closed head injuries, gunshot wounds, and multiple orthopedic trauma. The philosophy of the Trauma Center is to include early interdisciplinary rehabilitation. The physicians demand highly specialized knowledge and skills of all therapists before permitting their autonomous function within the Trauma Center. The position of lead therapist requires highly specialized knowledge and experience to groom and coordinate the activities of the other therapists assigned to the Trauma Center. The search for a new lead therapist, therefore, was broad and intense.

Because of the specific and high level of requirements for the position of lead therapist in the Trauma Center, the number of applicants was limited. The search committee, consisting of Ben Sawyer, director of rehabilitation, a physician from the Trauma Center and a therapist assigned to the Trauma Center (but not an applicant for the position), reviewed all the applications and interviewed the three most highly qualified candidates, either in person or by telephone conference call. The position was subsequently offered to and accepted by Henry Jackson, PT.

Mr. Jackson is 36 years old. He earned a Master of Science in Physiology and has 11 years experience as a physical therapist. For 8 years he worked in acute care hospitals, including a fair amount of time in intensive care units. For the past 3 years he was the chief physical therapist in the trauma center at a university-affiliated hospital in the North. He was strongly recommended by his department head and by the therapists and physicians in that trauma center. He demonstrated outstanding knowledge, skill, and patient interaction ability, in addition to being an extremely effective interdisciplinary team leader. Mr. Jackson chose to relocate because of the combination of the excellent reputation of Metropolitan Medical Center and his desire to be in a warmer climate, where he and his family could enjoy outdoor activities the year round.

Mr. Jackson arrived at Metropolitan Hospital, settled in quickly, and performed up to expectations. It was apparent that he was happy in his new environment and the department was happy with him. And then the bubble burst!

After Mr. Jackson was on the job about 6 weeks, Ms. Branch informed him that in 1 month he would have a team of two mid-stage students (one PT, one OT) for a 4-week clinical education assignment. This arrangement, made nearly a year ago, had been approved by Mr. Jackson's predecessor. After listening to Ms. Branch explain the arrangement, Mr. Jackson politely but firmly stated that he had no intention of accepting the students and suggested she assign them elsewhere. Ms. Branch countered by stating it was too late. The department had its full complement of clinical education students; therefore she "must insist" that he take the assigned students.

Mr. Jackson told Ms. Branch he regretted the situation, but a number of reasons compelled him to reject the student assignment. His reasons for refusal were (1) he considered patient care his primary responsibility, and he and his team were extremely busy; (2) on the basis of his past experience he believed that students lacked sufficient knowledge to function in the tense and demanding environment of a sophisticated trauma center; (3) though he expected and looked forward to clinical teaching, no one suggested to him that he would be expected to accept teams of mid-stage students; and (4) a 4-week assignment was too short to be of any significant value to any student. The only exception he would make would be a single physical therapy student in a final clinical education rotation who had prior work experience in a trauma setting. After further discussion between the two, Mr. Jackson refused to yield on his position. As a result, an angry Ms. Branch, who reports directly to the director of rehabilitation on matters pertaining to clinical education, immediately made an appointment to see Mr. Sawyer to discuss her problem.

When Mr. Sawyer and Ms. Branch met the following day, the latter had cooled off some. Nevertheless, she was still angry and resentful of the challenge to her authority as CCCE. Mr. Sawyer admitted discussing clinical education in general terms during the conference call interview with Mr. Jackson, but he recalled no mention of specific details such as teaching teams of students in the Trauma Center. Ms. Branch candidly admitted not having discussed that particular issue either. Mr. Sawyer procured a copy of the job description for Mr. Jackson's position and, though there was reference to clinical teaching, it was not specific. When asked if the students could be reassigned to another team, Ms. Branch replied that a full complement of students was already scheduled for the time period in question. In addition, the students and their faculty specifically requested the Trauma Center nearly a year ago because of the students' expressed interest. The coordination of assignments of teams of students from different schools is no easy task and permits limited flexibility. Ms. Branch added that the schools involved were among their oldest and most reliable affiliations and ones from which Metropolitan recruited heavily to fill vacant positions. For these reasons, Ms. Branch was reluctant to renege on this commitment. She concluded by asking, "What are you going to do about it?"

Complete Steps 1 to 3 of the problem-solving model.

Steps 3–5

Investigating, Analyzing, and Confirming the Problem

SCENARIO: CASE 8

HOW WILL YOU KNOW?
Writing Measurable Objectives

West River Rehabilitation Hospital (WRRH) is a comprehensive rehabilitation facility providing both in-house and out-patient services to the region it serves. It was recently acquired by Western Regional Health Systems (WRHS), a large, integrated health system based in a neighboring city. Senora Strong, director of speech and audiology, has been at WRRH for 6 years, the last 3 in her present capacity as director. Ms. Strong is able, enthusiastic, fair, and honest, and she possesses good interpersonal attitudes and skills. She is popular with her staff, other department heads, and higher administration. Her management style is participatory and flexible.

The speech and audiology department has been running smoothly. The staff is usually at full complement with a low turnover rate, and the department has never been significantly short-staffed. Under Ms. Strong's leadership there has been no evidence of friction among staff or with other departments or with the administration. The department has consistently operated with a respectable ratio of expenses-to-budget allocation.

With the purchase by WRHS, Tom Stancil resigned as president of WRRH and was immediately replaced by a new chief executive, Ms. Carol Yancey. Upon assuming the office of president, Ms. Yancey held a joint meeting of all department heads. She described her method and style of management, and she explained that WRHS's philosophy encouraged top management to establish broad organizational goals with input from the department level. All departments were expected to develop specific objectives compatible with and contributing to the broader goals of the organization. Ms. Yancey expressed the desire to become more familiar with the role and function of all the hospital's departments. Her first step would be to review the current objectives of each department. Therefore, she requested that each department submit objectives for the current fiscal year.

Ms. Strong was impressed by Ms. Yancey, and many of her initial fears about the acquisition by WRHS were subsiding. She confidently submitted the following objectives for the Speech and Audiology Department.

1. To provide high quality speech and audiology services
2. To function at a high level of efficiency
3. To operate fiscally within budget
4. To provide a high standard of clinical education for speech and audiology students
5. To provide opportunity for staff development

A week later Ms. Yancey invited Ms. Strong to meet and discuss these objectives. Ms. Yancey complimented Ms. Strong on her department, indicating that she based her comments on what she had heard from a variety of sources around the hospital. She then proceeded, however, to express her disappointment in the written departmental objectives. Although the objectives appeared admirable, they lacked specificity and were not measurable.

Ms. Yancey asked Ms. Strong, "With the exception of operation within the budget, how do you know if you have reached your objectives?" Ms. Strong was taken aback by the question and realized she did not have an adequate answer. Ms. Yancey suggested that Ms. Strong rewrite the departmental objectives in more specific and measurable terms and resubmit them within 2 weeks.

Step 1—Recognizing

Ms. Strong returned to her office to think about what had occurred. She recognized that she had a problem. This problem was different from most problems she encountered. In this case it was not a matter of making a choice, rather it was a matter of complying with a directive in a manner satisfactory to her administrator.

Step 2—Defining

As she sat in her office, she admitted to herself that the departmental objectives were vague and unmeasurable, but she also wondered, "How can I gather specific, measurable, and meaningful data about quality of service, efficiency, clinical education, and staff development?"

Step 3—Investigating

For help in answering this question, Ms. Strong turned to the rehabilitation management literature and several key manuals recommended by her management colleagues at other facilities.

Continue Ms. Strong's investigation of the characteristics of measurable behavioral objectives. Analyze her objectives in relation to the information you acquire through your investigation. Confirm the problem with the objectives as written and develop alternative objectives for the department that will enable Ms. Strong to determine whether the Speech and Audiology Department is attaining its goals.

SCENARIO: CASE 9

I DESERVE A MERIT INCREASE
Valuing Work Performance

Bella Vista Hospital is a large urban hospital with a rehabilitation department consisting of a budgeted staff of 50 therapists, 15 assistants, and a complement of support and clerical personnel. The organizational structure includes the director (Ms. Martinez); an assistant director (Mr. Thomas); 5 team leaders who supervise from 6 to 10 therapists each; and a number of specialists who conduct sport, industrial, hand, and back programs.

The hospital has a salary plan that provides for an annual cost-of-living increment for all employees and assigns each department additional funds equal to 4 percent of its payroll for discretionary allocation based on merit (defined as "exceeding job expectations"). Although the director has full authority to allocate merit increments, Ms. Martinez established a protocol for determination of merit raises (Table 1).

The work performance evaluation (WPE) for a team member is completed by the team leader and reviewed by the assistant director. The WPE ratings range from zero (fails to meet job expectations) to 5 (always exceeds job expectations). The items rated in the WPE for team therapists include the following:

TABLE 1
Protocol for Determination of Merit Raises

Position	Authority
Assistant director	Determined by the director
Team leaders	Recommended by assistant director and approved by the director
PT specialist	Joint determination by the director and assistant director
Team members	Recommended by team leader, approved by assistant director with final approval by the director.

1. Attendance
2. Punctuality
3. Professional knowledge
4. Professional skills
5. Patient documentation—timeliness/accuracy/clarity/thoroughness
6. External reports—timeliness/clarity/thoroughness
7. Billing/charge procedures—timeliness/accuracy
8. Patient rapport
9. Initiative
10. Responsibility
11. Supervisory skills

The process of work performance evaluation and determination of specific merit raises for the next fiscal year was completed, and each employee received an official notification of the raise he or she was to receive. On the second day following notification of merit awards, Rob Stone, a therapist assigned to team C, requested an appointment to meet with Ms. Martinez. The request was readily granted and the two agreed to meet early the next morning. Ms. Martinez was familiar with Mr. Stone, but as was her practice before private meetings with staff, she reviewed his employment folder. The contents of the folder revealed that Mr. Stone joined the department immediately upon graduation from school. He was now well into his fourth year of employment and his second year on team C. His performance ratings for the past 2 years were satisfactory, but not exemplary. There was no indication of any major criticism of his attitude or performance. Ms. Martinez did note, however, that on his most recent WPE he wrote under employee comments, "I do not believe these ratings accurately reflect my performance in a number of areas." She recalled reading that statement when she reviewed all the WPEs, and she now regretted not taking the opportunity to follow up and learn the basis of that statement. Her direct observation of Mr. Stone suggested a polite and personable young man who was popular with other members of his team and the department.

When Ms. Martinez and Mr. Stone met, he thanked her for agreeing to meet with him and indicated the purpose of the meeting was to "respectfully protest that for the second consecutive year I have received a less than fair work performance evaluation resulting in my not receiving any merit raise." He contended, that for reasons unknown to him, his team leader, Ms. Barnett, did not seem to like him or value his effort or performance. He was particularly disappointed in the latest WPE which, as he wrote on the form, failed to reflect his true performance.

Ms. Martinez asked why he came to her rather than to Mr. Thomas, the assistant director. Mr. Stone replied that since the normal procedure for work performance evaluations required Mr. Thomas' approval of Ms. Barnett's rating, he saw no point in going to him. Ms. Martinez, though not entirely pleased with that response, could understand Mr. Stone's reaction. She admitted to Mr. Stone that since her direct involvement in the determination of merit raises for team members was minimal, she could make no direct response at that time. However, she promised to look into the matter and to discuss it with Mr. Thomas. She also promised Mr. Stone she would get back to him as soon as possible.

Following Mr. Stone's departure, Ms. Martinez mentally reviewed the conversation and concluded that a problem existed and that it could not be left unattended. Although she had promised to speak to the assistant director, Ms. Martinez decided that before she did so she had best define the problem in a form that would suggest the kind of information to seek prior, during, and after that discussion. Ms. Martinez composed the following problem statement: "Is Mr. Stone justified in his allegation that recent WPEs do not accurately reflect his work performance, thus denying him a merit raise the past 2 years?" Ms. Martinez perceived her attempt to answer that question as a preliminary investigation which might help avoid a major confrontation.

Progress to Step 3 of the problem-solving model and identify the relevant information needed and the strategies to be employed in obtaining the information, without confronting the team leader.

SCENARIO: CASE 10

RIGHT-SIZING
Looking Ahead Through Retrenchment

State University Teaching Hospital (SUTH) is a large, comprehensive tertiary-care facility closely affiliated with the State University Medical School. Because it is partially subsidized by the state, the hospital operates under a mandate to accept and treat all patients, regardless of ability to pay. The mission statement of the hospital, as befits a university teaching hospital, emphasizes service, teaching, and research. Over the years the fiscal fortunes of the hospital fluctuated somewhat in response to the generosity of the state legislature, but on the whole the hospital fared well fiscally and counted on the legislature to be supportive of operational and capital needs. A number of developments, however, have caused great upheaval in the hospital's fiscal stability and the manner in which it does business.

One significant problem now affecting SUTH is the debt incurred for rapid capital expansion that took place a few years ago when interest rates were very high. The hospital received legislative approval to issue bonds to finance a number of expansion projects, and unfortunately, not all of the new projects progressed as anticipated. As a result, the cost of meeting the high interest payments on the bonds, in combination with the underutilization of the new projects, is a severe financial drag.

Another misfortune occurring almost in conjunction with the issuance of the hospital bonds was the erosion of the national and state economies. The state's finances were in such poor shape that the legislature, though reluctant to do so, significantly cut SUTH's budget in each of the past and current fiscal years, with little prospect for any applicable increase in the coming year.

A third major impact on SUTH's financial status and practice is the evolutionary change occurring in health delivery and reimbursement. The restrictive funding of Medicare and Medicaid, the dramatic growth of managed health care organizations in the state, and the increasingly complicated and restrictive payment policies of insurance companies all contribute to the need for SUTH to tighten its organizational belt and dramatically revise its way of doing business.

The top administrative officials of SUTH carefully collected and analyzed all the relevant fiscal data, including the best-informed estimate of state funding for the coming year, and determined that the hospital faced a deficit of more than $10 million. After further consideration of alternatives and strategies, the administrator, with the approval of the hospital's board of directors, decided that the best way to eliminate the deficit was to require all departments in the hospital to reduce their budgets for the next fiscal year by 10 percent of the current budget.

Rick Fallon, director of rehabilitation, has been a rehabilitation professional for more than 20 years. He has worked in a variety of settings and has 15 years experience as a department head. He has been in his present position for 10 years and is a dynamic and effective leader. Rick knew for some time that the hospital was in difficult financial straits and that there would be some cost-cutting measures taken. That knowledge had not prepared him, however, for the bombshell meeting of all department heads. Rick could hardly believe his ears when he learned of the decision regarding the 10 percent cut in all departments. During the ensuing discussion it was emphasized that the only restriction was that individual salaries could not be reduced, but other than that each department head could use his or her discretion in arriving at the revised budget. It was made emphatically clear that the decision was final and there were to be no exceptions. Rick retreated to his office, taking no consolation in the fact that he was not alone in having to cope with a most unpleasant development.

Rick could not help but reflect on his career, which had been highlighted by an era of continuous growth. As the head of three different departments, not only had he been permitted to expand the scope of those respective programs, he had been encouraged to do so! After 15 years of managing departments viewed as highly profitable revenue centers, he suddenly found himself as head of a cost center. Rick realized with dismay that he had to completely revise his way of thinking and his budgetary methods. He felt overwhelmed with the thought that after 15 years of progressive planning for growth, he now had to plan for a 10 percent cut. He had two immediate thoughts: "I have one monstrous problem on my hands" (Step 1—recognizing). "How in the world am I going to reduce my budget 10 percent?" (Step 2—defining).

Rick recognized that he had already completed the first two steps in problem solving and now thought about the next step (Step 3—investigating). It occurred to him that since he had never tackled a downsizing problem before, he might fail to identify all the information required to lead to a reasonable solution. Consequently, he invited his assistant director and supervisors to meet with him. He explained in detail the situation they faced and asked for their assistance in identifying the particular information they needed to proceed. He scheduled a brainstorming session for the next afternoon. He encouraged the group to list any idea that came to mind, without evaluative comments or discussion. The group constructed the following list of items in random sequence:

1. Exactly how much does the 10 percent come to in dollars?
2. What part of that amount is allocated to salaries?
3. We'll need a complete list of individual salaries.
4. What was our capital budget this year?
5. Do we have any capital needs for next year?
6. What about imminent plans of department personnel? Are any planning to relocate? Go to graduate school? Retire?
7. How about productivity rates of personnel?
8. Longevity in the department should be considered.
9. What about personal matters such as being the family breadwinner? Single person dependent on wages? Degree of flexibility in relocating? Other comparable employment opportunities in the immediate area for different personnel?
10. What about knowledge/skill requirements for specific department services? Are all of our specialty programs necessary? Are there activities presently performed by rehab that could be reassigned to another service?
11. What would be the impact on quality of care and/or personal needs if b.i.d. and t.i.d. services were reduced to once daily?
12. What effect will downsizing have on our clinical education program? Can we modify our clinical education program in any way to reduce our personnel needs and still comply with the teaching component of the hospital's mission statement?
13. Are there developments in medical care that may reduce or eliminate the need for rehab intervention: for example, shorter average length of stay (ALOS) in the hospital or better pre-op instruction by the surgeon's support staff?
14. Which rehab services have the greatest impact on ALOS?
15. Is there any way to reduce overhead costs?
16. Are there state or hospital personnel policies that govern termination of employees in the case of fiscal exigency?
17. Is this downsizing viewed as permanent right-sizing for the medical center's future needs or as a temporary stall?

The assembled group was somewhat daunted by the wide diversity of information they needed. They agreed that the separate items needed to be organized or categorized into homogeneous groupings to enhance the efficiency and thoroughness of data gathering. They also recognized that the answers to some questions determined the relevance of the answers to others.

Categorize and reorder the questions in a manner that will expedite Step 3—investigating.

SCENARIO: CASE 11

BIAS AND PREJUDICE
Understanding Behavior

Sunrise Manor is a 200-bed nursing home, with 100 beds devoted to subacute care, 75 beds to intermediate nursing care, and 25 beds reserved for custodial care. Sunrise Manor is recognized by physicians and other health professionals as a progressive nursing facility with high standards. It provides a comprehensive range of services, and its personnel traditionally demonstrate concern for, and conscientious treatment of, the home's clients.

The Rehabilitation Department, though not large, is top quality, emphasizing a preventive approach with those occupying custodial and intermediate beds and a rehabilitation approach for patients who require subacute care. The facility consistently demonstrates an exceptional record of goal attainment by patients and a history of early discharge to the home environment.

The director of rehabilitation at Sunrise Manor for the past 3 years has been Angela Morelli, OTR/L. Before coming to Sunrise Manor she worked for several years in a small community hospital and then in a regional rehabilitation center. She applied for and accepted her present position because she particularly enjoyed working with older individuals. She was offered the position because of strong references that cited her concern for quality of care and her outstanding ability to motivate older patients with a combination of humor, charm, and patience. Since her earliest days at Sunrise Manor, Ms. Morelli has earned the respect and confidence of the administration, her staff, and other facility personnel, as well as the gratitude of many patients and their families.

The rehab department, in addition to Ms. Morelli, includes two physical therapists (PT), two physical therapist assistants (PTA), one other occupational therapist (OT), and two rehabilitation aides. One of the PTs, Sandy Bridges, has been in the department for 2 years, following 3 years employment in a general hospital. Jean Harris, the other PT, just joined the department following her graduation from school. She had excellent grades and strong recommendations from academic and clinical faculty. The remaining staff have been at Sunrise Manor from 1 to 8 years and all clearly reflected joy in their work and loyalty to Ms. Morelli and the organization.

Ms. Morelli generally is not a believer in close "over the shoulder" supervision, and in her present situation it is unnecessary because of the trust her staff has earned. The exceptions are when one of the staff requests observation and feedback and when there is an addition to the staff. She feels a responsibility to keep a close eye on new personnel, particularly if they are inexperienced.

By the completion of Ms. Harris's first month at Sunrise Manor, Ms. Morelli was very pleased. Ms. Harris impressed her as being bright, confident, independent but willing to seek and accept advice, hardworking, and good with patients. Her observations were seconded by other staff who worked in close proximity from time to time. As a consequence of this unanimous positive appraisal of Ms. Harris, Ms. Morelli eased the reins of supervision and spent less time observing her in action.

Over the next several months things seemed to be going smoothly. The only discordant notes came sporadically and from different directions. The first of these was from one of the PTAs who commented that Ms. Harris seemed to be "a bit rough on Mr. Brown this morning." The second was from the activities director who asked how she liked Ms. Harris. After responding, Ms. Morelli asked if there was some reason for asking the question, to which the activities director reported having observed Ms. Harris being impatient and rude with a patient. Not too many days later Ms. Bridges reluctantly admitted she happened to be nearby while Ms. Harris was treating Ms. Crump and was disturbed at the manner in which Ms. Harris treated her patient. Ms. Bridges indicated that the PT treatment was less than thorough and that Ms. Harris' attitude toward Ms. Crump was inexcusably rude.

Ms. Morelli was not pleased to hear the three disparaging remarks about Ms. Harris. The reported behavior was not in character with the enthusiastic young PT she had observed closely just 2 months ago, yet she had sufficient trust and confidence in her staff and in the activities director to feel the need to follow up on the allegations. To that end Ms. Morelli made a concerted effort to observe Ms. Harris as inconspicuously as possible. Because of her own caseload Ms. Morelli could spend only limited time observing Ms. Harris. For the first few days she observed no behavior that would support the allegations. On the third day Ms. Morelli was sufficiently close to hear and observe Ms. Harris treating Ms. Crump in a far from professional manner. To her dismay, Ms. Morelli had to classify the behavior as rude and abusive, and consistent with the allegations previously lodged against Ms. Harris.

Later that day Ms. Morelli sat in her office and mentally reviewed the day's disturbing development. She found it hard to accept Ms. Harris's abusive behavior but could not escape her own direct observation, nor could she avoid the obvious fact that this was not the first such incident. As she reviewed the incident, she redirected her focus to the patient. Ms. Crump had Alzheimer's disease, resulting in a very short memory span and little motivation to perform her exercise regimen. Ms. Morelli began to wonder about the other patients allegedly mistreated by Ms. Harris. She went to the patient files for information on the three individuals to whom Ms. Harris had been rude. Ms. Morelli discovered that each of the three was diagnosed as having Alzheimer's disease and each presented memory and motivation symptoms similar to Ms. Crump's!

Ms. Morelli appreciated the fact that many individuals with Alzheimer's disease can be trying and that treating them demands patience of the therapist. She believed that she had identified the common thread and cause of Ms. Harris's uncharacteristic behavior. However, there remained the possibility of mere coincidence. Ms. Morelli recognized a problem: "How do I confirm the suspicion that Ms. Harris has an attitudinal bias against patients with Alzheimer's disease?"

Ms. Morelli, in progressing to the investigative phase of problem solving, quickly realized that there was not much information to gather; she already had all the information that existed, three remarks by different individuals and her own direct observation. She believed the best source of information was Ms. Harris and decided to approach her directly. In an effort to minimize the formality and potential threat of a one-on-one meeting, Ms. Morelli invited Ms. Harris to the snack bar and, over a cup of coffee, tactfully but directly raised the issue of the treatment of certain patients.

Ms. Harris made no effort to deny the allegation. Rather, she apologized and said she simply could not help it. She revealed that she had a grandmother who had Alzheimer's disease and who had lived with her family the last 10 years of her life, as she steadily deteriorated in function and intellect.

Ms. Harris related that as a young girl she had to help care for her grandmother, feeding her and assisting with hygiene. She said she had loved her grandmother, but she was left with many unpleasant memories that are revived when working with recalcitrant patients with the same affliction. She concluded that even though she knew better intellectually, she nevertheless could not always control her emotions and at times lost her patience. Ms. Morelli thanked her for her honesty and then asked why she chose to work in the type of setting in which there were likely to be patients with Alzheimer's disease. Ms. Harris responded that she generally liked elderly persons, she wanted to work in that particular geographic location, the pay and benefits were good, she had heard many positive things about Ms. Morelli,and she had truly believed she could overcome the unpleasant experiences of the past. Ms. Morelli again thanked Ms. Harris for her candor and indicated she wanted a few days to think about the matter before meeting with her to discuss the future.

Ms. Morelli had gained the additional information she felt she needed, and after careful analysis of all the information, she determined that the original problem statement was no longer relevant and that she had a new problem. After a period of deliberation Ms. Morelli rephrased her problem: "Ms. Harris has an admitted attitudinal bias against patients with Alzheimer's disease. What should I do about it?"

What new information is required because of the revised problem statement? How might Ms. Morelli proceed with her investigation and analysis before confirming her revised problem statement? Identify alternatives that might evolve from this new information.

SCENARIO: CASE 12

THE ULTIMATUM
The Value of an Individual to the Organization

Progressive Hospital is a tertiary-care hospital with 500 beds, including a 25-bed rehabilitation unit. The facility is well organized with clearly stated policies to serve as guidelines and controls for departmental managers, who are afforded a generous amount of latitude and flexibility within the stated administrative guidelines.

Among the management prerogatives available to all department heads is the authority to independently determine salaries and salary increments for all departmental personnel, with the following limitations:

1. The total payroll must remain within the amount officially budgeted for the fiscal year.
2. The maximum salary increment that can be awarded to any individual in one year is 15 percent, unless the individual has received an approved formal promotion.

For the past 2 years salary increments have averaged 8 percent, with a range of 3 to 12 percent.

The Physical Therapy Department of Progressive Hospital numbers about 30 PTs, 10 PTAs, and numerous other support personnel. Figure 2 is a diagram of the organizational structure of the department.

Each of the teams is organized by the type of caseload or special services provided, such as orthopedic outpatient and sports, ICU-cardipulmonary, etc. The team leaders, in addition to providing direct patient care, have major supervisory and staff development responsibilities. Promotion to the position of team leader is based on a combination of administrative skill and expertise in the respective specialty area.

As the scenario unfolds, it is late in the fiscal year. Ms. Jones, the director of physical therapy, has reviewed the work performance evaluations (WPE) of all staff and has reviewed team performance in efficiency, performance improvement, and attainment of annual objectives. She is now in the final stages of budget preparation for the coming fiscal year, including the determination of merit increments. In reviewing team and individual performance, Ms. Jones observed that for the third con-

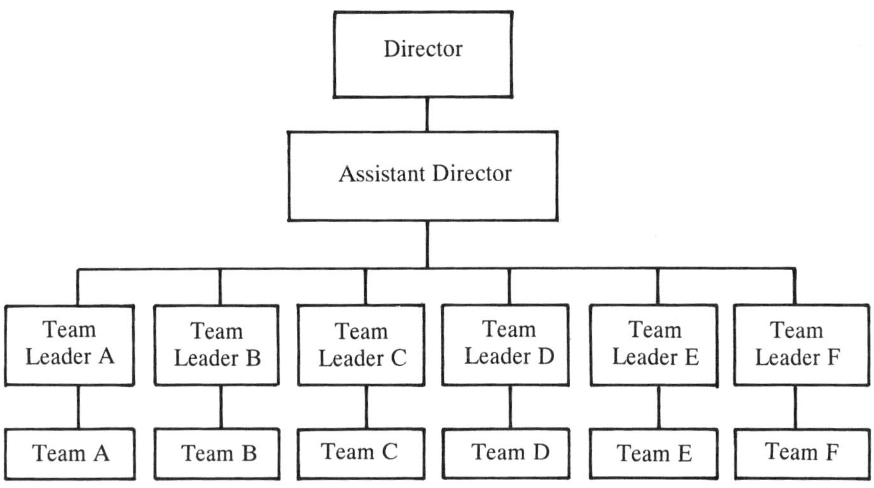

FIGURE 2

secutive year team leader A had scored appreciably higher on her WPE than any of her colleagues.

Unfortunately for the director, her budget thoughts and plans were interrupted by team leader A, who unexpectedly announced that another physical therapy service in the area has offered her a similar position with a salary 25 percent higher than her present salary. Team leader A indicated that she enjoys her work and the association with the director and her department colleagues. She further expressed a desire to remain at Progressive Hospital, however, she found it difficult to ignore a 25 percent pay differential. Team leader A indicated a willingness to remain in her present position if Ms. Jones was willing to provide her the maximum merit increment of 15 percent in the coming fiscal year. Ms. Jones, who has known team leader A for 5 years and has complete faith in her integrity, has no doubt as to the authenticity of the offer from the other organization, nor does she have any doubt that team leader A will leave if offered anything less than the maximum increment allowed. Ms. Jones thanked team leader A for her offer and indicated she would consider it and give her a response within a few days.

Following the departure of team leader A, Ms. Jones gave thought to her situation and quickly recognized the possibility of major repercussions whatever decision she made. She also recognized immediately that this was not a decision that could be made by emotion, loyalty, or superficial thinking. With those thoughts in mind, Ms. Jones decided to apply a problem-solving approach to her dilemma. Step 1 (Recognizing) was quickly accomplished in that she was aware of the need to make a decision because of the ultimatum presented by team leader A and because of the approaching deadline for submission of a proposed budget. Step 2 (Defining) also was quickly completed by stating the problem as, "Do I agree to team leader A's demand for a 15 percent pay increment or do I refuse, knowing she will leave?"

Step 3 (Investigating) requires the gathering and organizing of relevant information.

Determine what information should be sought, and organize your anticipated responses in a manner that will assist you in proceeding through Steps 4 to 10.

SCENARIO: CASE 13

KEEPING THE LID ON IT
Coping With Dramatic and Rapid Change

Jamie Sawyer, MS, PT, has been the director of physical therapy at Yancey River Memorial Hospital for 12 years. Yancey River Memorial is a small community hospital nestled in the Appalachian mountains. Although rural by most measures, the city of Yancey River is sufficiently large to offer a bit of culture and urban attractiveness. Located near some of the most exclusive ski resorts in the East, it attracts businesses and activities that cater to a cosmopolitan crowd. The surrounding panorama is breathtaking, and just beyond the immediate area of the city and the slopes, real estate is reasonable, even for a young professional with a modest income.

Yancey River Memorial boasts about the quality of its health care. The staff takes a personal interest in patients and their problems. Because of the attractiveness of the location, Yancey River attracts many talented young physicians and other health professionals eager to provide high-quality care without the usual hassles of a major medical center. Yancey River has its share of problems related to shortened lengths of stay dictated by insurance carriers and slowed and limited reimbursement, but it is generally faring well. Its success can be attributed to its high standards, the lack of geographic competition from other hospitals, and a generous endowment by the city's original founder, who made his fortune in bituminous coal.

Two years ago Ms. Sawyer proposed to the administration that the Department of Physical Therapy, which included four physical therapists, an aide, and a secretary/receptionist, be expanded to include occupational therapy and speech and language pathology. She suggested that the services be reorganized under a collective department of rehabilitation. The recommendation was well supported in theory and by data gathered by Ms. Sawyer. Until this time the limited occupational and speech therapy services available at the hospital were provided under contract by a major national rehabilitation corporation at a rather hefty hourly fee. Through her contact in her own professional association and her recent work with the TriAlliance, a coalition of the occupational, physical, and speech/language professional associations in the state, Ms. Sawyer was confident about her ability to attract occupational therapists and speech pathologists to Yancey River. Employment of their own staff would substantially reduce the cost of occupational and speech therapy services and probably result in increased referrals and improved services for patients.

Administration agreed with her assessment and approved the change. Ms. Sawyer was correct in her assessment, and her predictions came true. Today, in addition to her original staff, she employes three occupational therapists and two speech/language pathologists, and she is contemplating a request to add both a physical therapist assistant and an occupational therapy assistant to the staff. She appointed a supervisor for each of the three services (OT, PT, and SP/L) and has been pleased about how well this core supervisory group has worked collaboratively for the well-being of the entire department.

Ms. Sawyer recognizes that growth has occurred very quickly over the past 2 years and that the staff is showing signs of the resulting stress. The major concern is the failure of the administration's space allocations to keep pace with the department's rapid growth. Tensions over personal and professional work space are high. Scheduling of patients in the department has become difficult as therapists from all three services vie for the same space. Staff are frequently abrupt with one another when work space is limited for writing notes and completing charge slips at the end of the day. These unpleasantries are quickly forgotten, however, and Ms. Sawyer is proud of the way her staff has adapted.

Ms. Sawyer has been equally pleased with her working relationship with Mr. Stanley, the vice president for operations to whom she reports. Mr. Stanley has also been at Yancey River for many years and has always supported Ms. Sawyer and trusted her judgment in the operation of the department. He was most supportive during the years she was enrolled part-time in a graduate program in health administration. He was flexible about providing administrative leave for some daytime classes, and he approved reimbursement for 60 percent of the program's tuition and fees. Ms. Sawyer recalls that those were difficult years, requiring many long and odd hours to keep up with both school and her administrative responsibilities at the hospital. She recognizes the value of her degree, however, and is glad she had the tenacity to stick it out.

Nothing in Ms. Sawyer's graduate program prepared her for the news she received at the department director's meeting that afternoon. Yancey River had been acquired by a large health-care conglomerate. The deal was finalized and made public that morning. It is now one of many small community hospitals in a chain along the East Coast that will be networked with larger tertiary hospitals, subacute centers, and home-health agencies. The philosophy of the new corporation is quite different from that of the local administration. Several changes have already been made in administrative staff. The former president and chief executive officer has been replaced by a corporate shining star, Noel Robinson. Several of the vice presidents have also been replaced, including Mr. Stanley. His desk is cleaned out, and he is already gone, without the opportunity even to say good-bye.

Each of the department directors, including Ms. Sawyer, was handed a new organizational chart and a proposed skeleton plan for operations. Ms. Sawyer recognized the plan as the patient-focused care model she had read about in her professional journal last month. She regrets her smugness at thinking it would never happen at Yancey River and wished she had saved the journal.

As Ms. Robinson explained the plan, each department director was assigned to an interdisciplinary planning team. The responsibility for working out the details and managing the transition was assigned to these planning teams. The stated goal is for the transition to be complete within 12 months. The administration is prepared to allow for some flexibility in the plan based on the recommendations of the planning teams, but the overall plan for patient-focused care and decentralization of departments is clearly not negotiable.

Scanning the proposal, Ms. Sawyer immediately realized that her department was marked for decentralization. Therapist positions were reassigned to interdisciplinary patient-care teams on the various patient-care units. The patient-care units were to be reorganized according to diagnosis and level of acuity, and the teams would share responsibility for meeting the patients' needs. Staff would be cross-trained in common patient-care procedures to increase efficiency.

Ms. Sawyer's position was reclassified as coordinator of ancillary care services, and she would now be responsible for respiratory therapy and therapeutic recreation services as well as physical, occupational, and speech therapy. The positions of the previous directors of these two services were slated for elimination sometime during the transition period. Ms. Sawyer will continue to have responsibility for the hiring and firing of staff in her assigned services and for monitoring performance and quality indicators. Obviously she will have to collaborate closely with nursing and the other disciplines to fulfill these responsibilities successfully. She now answers to the vice president for patient care, the previous director of nursing. Each of the therapists will answer directly to the unit nurse regarding patient care, scheduling, and daily activities.

The new administration presented a carefully prepared videotape and handed out supporting materials to explain the reorganization and the success of similar reorganizations at sister hospitals in the network. Ms. Robinson provided impressive documentation about efficiency and cost saving at hospitals that had made this transition several years ago. Also included were statements from patients, medical and professional staff, and managers at these other facilities regarding improved satisfaction and quality of services.

As the department directors left the meeting in shock, Ms. Sawyer wondered how to communicate this information to her staff. By the time she reached her office she realized this was no longer a concern. The hospital grapevine had outdone itself. They already knew. She was inundated with questions and concerns about what would happen next, who would be terminated, and how did the hospital possibly expect to save money if therapists were going to be expected to change linens and empty bedpans. Emotions were running high. Ms. Sawyer listened to their concerns and tried to reassure them that the transition would not be complete for another year. She informed them of her assignment to a transition planning team and committed herself to representing them well in the planning process. She suggested they schedule a special staff meeting for the first day of the next week to discuss the matter. This would give her time to review the materials provided by the administration and to collect her own thoughts.

Ms. Sawyer recognized that there was a problem, but she was unclear about how to define the problem in a manner that would assist her in formulating a course of action. In the security of her own office with the door closed, Ms. Sawyer tried to sort through feelings of shock and uncertainty. She was cognizant of her own fears about what these changes would mean for her personally, and she appreciated the fear that her staff was experiencing. She perused the "Positions Available" section of the current professional newsletter. She was not sure if she was more concerned about the implications of change for the hospital or the burden of leadership through the transition period. Ms. Robinson had been very convincing, and in spite of her loyalty to Mr. Stanley, she was intrigued by the opportunity to work with a fast-track administrator like Ms. Robinson. She also felt considerable loyalty to her staff and ownership in the quality of rehabilitation services to be provided under any model of service delivery.

After some consideration, Ms. Sawyer realized that what she was facing was not a "problem" per se, but a whopping "opportunity." It all boiled down to one question, "How do I successfully manage change of this magnitude?" She began developing a list of sources of information and resources that might be helpful in developing potential strategies. She started by listing the journal article she had inadvertently tossed away.

Where else might Ms. Sawyer turn for help or to gather additional information?

SCENARIO: CASE 14

VIVE LA DIFFÉRENCE!
Requirements Versus Preferences

Crocker County encompasses an area of about 800 square miles, roughly 35 miles north to south and 25 miles east to west. It is primarily an agricultural region, but it does include several large towns within its borders, including the county capital of Central City with a population of about 50,000. In addition to being the home of the county government offices, it is the location of the Crocker County Home Health Agency (CCHHA).

The CCHHA, like many of its counterparts, has grown significantly in recent years because of reduced hospital stays, resulting in an increased demand for home services. Jim Walsh, the director of rehabilitation, has seen his staff expand from three full-time-equivalent (FTE) physical therapists to eight FTE physical therapists, five FTE occupational therapists, and two FTE speech pathologists. The staff includes 10 full-time and 12 part-time or contract employees. Paralleling this growth is the inevitable expansion of management responsibilities and the inability of Mr. Walsh to keep up with everything.

Mr. Walsh recognized his inability to discharge his administrative activities with efficiency and effectiveness and, after much thought and discussion with others, decided to create a position of assistant director to handle many of the day-to-day activities. Walsh's request and job description were approved by the administrator, and both agreed that the position should be advertised internally and appointment to the position made from among current staff.

Among the components of the now-official job description was a section labeled "Job Qualifications," with the following entries:

1. State licensure as an occupational therapist, physical therapist, or speech pathologist
2. Minimum of 3 years professional experience in home health care
3. Minimum of 1 year supervisory or management experience
4. Ability to communicate effectively orally and in writing
5. Job performance demonstrating good organization and skill in working with others

Of the 10 therapists employed full-time, 2 submitted applications for the new position. None of the part-time staff expressed an interest in the position. The two applicants were Ed White, PT, and Ruth Hayes, OTR/L. Mr. White has 7 years experience as a PT, including the last 3 with CCHHA. Before coming to CCHHA, Mr. White worked for 2 years as a team leader in a large teaching hospital. Ms. Hayes has 4 years experience as an OT in home health care, with the last year and a half at CCHHA. Other than clinical supervision of OT assistants, Ms. Hayes has no formal supervisory or management experience.

After the deadline for applications had passed, Mr. Walsh reviewed the two applications with genuine concern. On the basis of credentials, Mr. White appeared to be the clear choice for the promotion. He had 3 more years of experience and 2 years of supervisory experience. Although Ms. Hayes had 1 additional year of experience in home health care, she had no supervisory experience. However, direct observation and informal reports strongly suggested that Mr. White, although a very competent therapist, was more of an individualist than a team player.

Mr. Walsh's personal observations of Mr. White's job performance and the periodic complaints of other members of the staff relating to his work attitudes and interpersonal skills showed that Mr. White had a history of concern only for his personal convenience and preferred manner of doing things. He never offered to adjust his schedule to assist his colleagues with problems or unexpected changes. In addition, he was perceived as being very opinionated and reluctant to consider other views or methods. Although he was not antisocial or openly disruptive of organizational policies and procedures, he not infrequently was very abrupt or caustic in his communication with colleagues. He was perceived as being impatient and often short-tempered when things did not go as expected. And finally, although Mr. Walsh considered Mr. White conscientious and hardworking, he did not regard him as a well-organized individual.

Conversely, Ms. Hayes was very popular among her peers and other agency personnel. She was always polite, tactful, and considerate of others, and she was a very effective communicator. In terms of organizational skill, communication, and interpersonal relations, there was no question in Mr. Walsh's mind that Ms. Hayes was the superior candidate for the newly created position.

It may be useful for Mr. Walsh to proceed through the first four steps of the problem-solving model.

Step 1—Recognizing

Is there a problem that requires resolution? Yes!

Step 2—Defining

Which of the two official candidates should I select to be the assistant director?

Step 3—Investigating

The information pertaining to the credentials and performance of the candidates is readily available from the preceding discussion.

Step 4—Analyzing

Ms. Hayes best demonstrates those qualities perceived to be necessary for success as the assistant director. However, she does not meet the stipulated qualification of 1 year supervisory experience.

Mr. Walsh has now reached Step 5, where he must confirm or redefine the problem.

How would you proceed?

Steps 6–7

Developing Alternative Strategies and Identifying the Positive and Negative Factors of Each

SCENARIO: CASE 15

MANAGING INVENTORY
At What Cost?

Sam Palermo and Rob Keene are partners and co-owners of a physical therapy out-patient clinic. Sam and Rob are very compatible as friends and entrepreneurs. They take pleasure and pride in the success and growth of their venture over the past 5 years. Both of the men, in addition to being physical therapists, are certified athletic trainers. From the beginning the practice emphasized the treatment of orthopedic and sports-related problems.

The practice, which was successful from the start, continued to grow, and they moved from their original rented location 2 years ago to a new free-standing building that they designed and built to their specifications. The building is spacious, nicely decorated, and well equipped. Last year they merged with a national network of physical therapy practices and expanded their services to include wellness and return-to-work programs. They are optimistic about their future security.

In addition to themselves, Sam and Rob employ three physical therapists, two physical therapist assistants, one aide, one bookkeeper, and one secretary/receptionist. Sam and Rob routinely meet early each Tuesday morning to discuss developments and problems and to touch base on their respective progress on major planning activities. On this particular Tuesday morning, after all other items on their informal agenda had been cleared, Sam asked Rob if he had noticed that the monthly towel inventory showed a decrease in the total number of bath towels for the past 3 months? The loss through attrition had previously been constant at two or three towels a month. The number of missing towels the past 3 months had risen to four or five. Since the replacement cost of each terry cloth towel was $8, this represented a loss of up to $40 per month, or $16 per month more than had been the norm. Although $40 per month represents an almost infinitesimal part of their monthly revenues, as good businessmen they were concerned.

Sam and Rob discussed the matter and agreed that these increased losses should not be casually ignored. They reviewed (1) their monthly inventory process, conducted by the aide the first thing in the morning on the first workday of the month; (2) the procedure for counting towels at the time of the laundry service's pickup and delivery, also performed by the aide; and (3) the documentation procedure for the discard of worn-out towels. There had been no changes in any of the procedures for more than a year.

The partners turned their attention to their personnel. The only recent additions were one physical therapist and one physical therapist assistant, both of whom were employed 6 months ago. The aide responsible for the towel inventory and exchange with the laundry service was a trusted employee who had been working for them for more than 3 years. Neither Sam nor Rob had any indication that other items were disappearing, and neither could identify a reason for suspicion of any of the employees. The only other persons who entered the premises with any regularity were the patients (always more than 60 per day) and the Joneses, a husband and wife team who had been doing an excellent job of cleaning their building at a reasonable price for the past 2 years. The Joneses were recommended to them as being impeccably honest, and there had never been any reason to suspect them of any theft, however minor.

After reviewing procedures and personnel, Sam asked Rob, "What can we do about the additional losses?"

Develop a list of possible actions. Identity the positive and negative factors associated with each.

SCENARIO: CASE 16

ALLOCATION OF MERIT INCREMENTS
Values in Work Performance

Mr. Tom Crown is the director of rehabilitation at City Hospital, heading a department that includes an assistant director, 3 supervisors, 24 senior and staff therapists, and a variety of support personnel. Mr. Crown recently received notification about preparation of a proposed budget for the next fiscal year, including the designation of salary increments in accordance with institutional policy. The hospital's salary-increment policy gives all employees an automatic increment of 3 percent; in addition, the hospital allocates a pool of funds equal to 5 percent of the total of eligible salaries segregated by job classification (i.e., supervisors, staff therapists) to each department for merit raises. The director of each department awards these funds based on meritorious service and work performance evaluations. The funds may not be redistributed across job classifications nor used for any purpose other than merit raises. There is provision for a department head to award up to 10 percent to any individual as long as the total of all merit awards does not exceed the total amount of the pool. This is Mr. Crown's first opportunity to determine merit increments, since he assumed his present position after the beginning of the current fiscal year.

In addition to the director and assistant director, the department has three services, each consisting of a supervisor, a senior therapist, five to seven staff therapists, and two therapist assistants. Each supervisor completes biannual work performance evaluations (WPEs) for all service members. The director and assistant director perform joint evaluations of the three supervisors. Because this was his first attempt at determining merit awards and also because of his participatory management style, Mr. Crown reviewed the staff WPEs with each supervisor and with the assistant director to determine merit awards. Mr. Crown then deliberated with his assistant director to determine merit awards for the three supervisors.

The first step in the deliberation concerning merit increments for the supervisors was a review of their WPEs. The WPE document employed was fairly sophisticated with a clearly defined numerical rating key and a comprehensive list of items to be rated. The items rated were consistent with the principal activities of the supervisors and were derived from the job description. In addition, space was provided for supporting and clarifying comments or for indication of specific items in need of remediation.

The scores on the respective WPEs strongly suggested that supervisor "A" had performed at the highest level, with supervisor "C" appreciably lower. The performance rating of supervisor "B" fell between the two, clearly below supervisor "A," but just as clearly above supervisor "C."

Mr. Crown and his assistant director realized that numbers alone sometimes fail to reveal the entire story. Consequently, they discussed the three supervisors in terms of subjective as well as objective information.

Both agreed on the following points:

1. Of the three supervisors, "A" demonstrated the most innate talent for the position, but realizes less of her vast potential than the others.
2. "C" has been a supervisor for less than 2 years, whereas the other two have been in their present positions about 4 years each.
3. For perceived effort and realization of potential, "C" received the highest rating, with "B" next.
4. For team productivity and accomplishment, the "A" team received ratings far above the other two, with the "B" team next.
5. Each of the supervisors is loyal to the organization and its leaders.
6. None of the supervisors was guilty of any serious behavioral or attitudinal problems or deficits.

The annual salaries of the supervisors are

"A"	$ 45,000
"B"	43,000
"C"	40,000
Total salaries	$128,000
Multiplied by 5 percent	.05
Supervisor merit pool	$ 6,400

Mr. Crown must make a decision.

What options might Mr. Crown and his assistant consider for allocation of merit increments? Which supervisor(s) should receive a merit increment and what should be the amount(s) awarded? What are the positive and negative factors associated with the various options you identify?

SCENARIO: CASE 17

OH! THE FRUSTRATION OF IT ALL
The Value of Coalitions for Promoting Change

New to Regional Rehabilitation Center (RRC) and to the job of director of occupational therapy, Nell Bryant, OTR/L believed it was important for her to orient herself as to the facility and key personnel with whom she expected to interact (Fig. 3). Ms. Bryant spent her first several weeks meeting with the occupational therapy (OT) staff individually, as teams, and as a group; meeting with key personnel in other departments; walking around the center, introducing herself to personnel she encountered; and observing her staff in all phases of the department's operations.

Ms. Bryant's individual and group meetings with OT personnel reflected a generally positive attitude with one exception. Concerns were expressed about the quality of nursing care at RRC. The OT staff alleged that nursing personnel were deficient in (1) encouraging patients to practice ADL functions, (2) following up on positioning and the use of splints or other adaptive equipment, and (3) performing passive range of motion (PROM). Ms. Bryant, in her travels about the center, suspected the same deficiencies. After her staff complained, she visited several units again, and to her dismay confirmed the staff's allegations. She knew from years of experience that such deficiencies impede patient progress and may result in patient loss of function. She was very concerned.

Ms. Bryant decided to focus on the problem at her next departmental meeting. As the discussion progressed, she was disturbed to hear the department veterans state that the problem was an old and continuous one. The nursing staff simply ignored

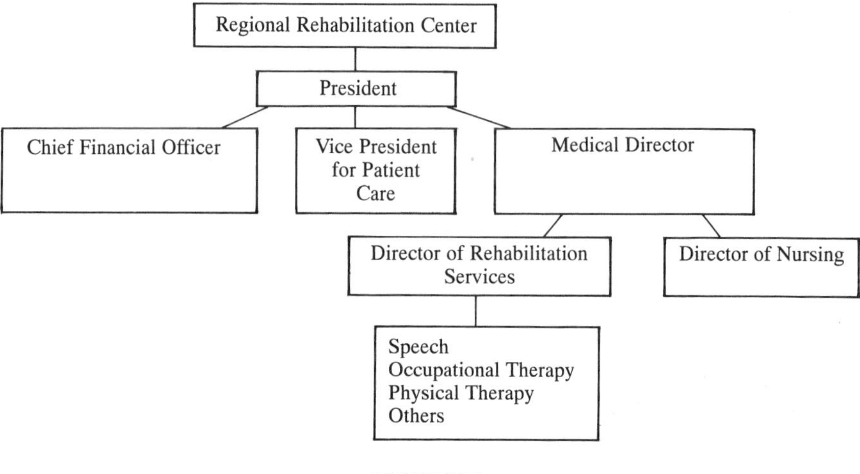

FIGURE 3

OTs' pleas for better service for their patients. If the OTs complained too much or too loudly, the nursing staff retaliated with double-scheduling, tardiness for OT appointments, and other annoying actions. Ms. Bryant's staff indicated that the customary complaint process was for a complaint or request to be made to the unit nurse. The unit nurse was to pass it along to the nursing supervisor, who then directed the complaint or request to the director of nursing. No discernible change in behavior had been noted in the past as a result of this complaint process.

Because of this history, and because she preferred to promote a positive atmosphere of teamwork with other services, Ms. Bryant asked her staff to try another approach. She suggested they make a concerted effort to develop rapport with the nursing service, citing the old adage of "attracting more flies with honey than with vinegar." She asked her staff to eliminate complaints, no matter how justified, and to try to be as friendly as possible with nursing staff. She personally went out of her way to be friendly with the nursing staff and their supervisors.

The response to the friendly overtures of the OT staff and Ms. Bryant was cool at best. The nursing staff was perhaps even more derelict in their responsibilities. Ms. Bryant, therefore, tried another strategy. She invited Ms. Hurley, director of nursing, to lunch and tried to discuss the issues in an informal and less confrontational setting. Ms. Hurley's attitude remained cool and defensive. She concluded the discussion by stating that she had limited staff and her nurses could not do all the things expected of them. The issues of concern to OT were hardly at the top of their list of priorities and by necessity were frequently ignored. Ms. Bryant expressed understanding of Ms. Hurley's situation. She asked if she could meet in a group session with Ms. Hurley and her supervisors to try to find some way to address these concerns despite the limitations. Ms. Hurley responded with, "No, we will not waste any more of our time."

Although they had refrained from lodging complaints, Ms. Bryant and her OT staff conscientiously documented nursing deficiencies in patient care. Ms. Bryant catalogued the more serious complaints and submitted them in her regular written reports to Mr. Bacon, the director of rehabilitation services. When Mr. Bacon failed to respond to her complaints within a reasonable period of time, Ms. Bryant decided to voice her concerns to him directly at his next meeting of department heads. When she did, the director of physical therapy was quick to support Ms. Bryant's allegations. Mr. Bacon indicated that he had no reason to doubt the allegations and reluctantly agreed to approach Ms. Hurley about them. He predicted that nothing would change.

After another month with no noticeable change in the quality of nursing care, Ms. Bryant again raised her concerns at the next meeting of department heads. Mr. Bacon had talked with Ms. Hurley but to no avail. Ms. Bryant wanted to abide by the administrative chain of command; therefore, she requested Mr. Bacon's permission to approach Dr. Earley, the medical director, to discuss these concerns. Mr. Bacon denied the request. Ms. Bryant was angry and frustrated.

Over the next several weeks several incidents occurred that further evidenced the less than adequate care provided by the nursing staff. A teenage boy with quadriplegia developed two decubitus ulcers, directly attributable to the fact he was not turned in bed as frequently as prescribed. Two other patients were losing passive range of motion. Both reported they had received no PROM activity on the ward as prescribed, despite their personal requests of nurses. A patient who had learned to use adapted eating utensils was not given the opportunity to practice with them on his unit, thus retarding his progression to independence. When Ms. Bryant learned of these incidents from her angry staff, her own level of anger and frustration was rekindled. She walked to the nursing station and proceeded to castigate the nursing staff and the supervisor for their negligence.

Within a few hours Mr. Bacon summoned Ms. Bryant to his office. He reported that Ms. Hurley had filed a formal complaint against Ms. Bryant, and he reprimanded her for "exceeding her authority and deviating from normal lines of communication." He told her he would not tolerate such behavior. Ms. Bryant left Mr. Bacon's office and went directly to the office of Mr. Sharpe, the vice president for patient care. He granted her an audience but, as she began to relate the situation, he cut her off and told her to go through the proper channels if she had a complaint. Ms. Bryant returned to her office, locked the door, and asked herself, "What now?"

Ms. Bryant's mind was a whirl. She concurrently considered resigning, accepting the status quo, and new strategies to effect a positive change. After she calmed down and managed to get her adrenaline under control, she organized her thoughts. She realized she had a serious problem. She cleared her desk, pulled out a blank tablet and began the process of problem solving.

Ms. Bryant had sufficient insight to appreciate that her initial thoughts covered a wide and disparate range. She tried to focus on the problem. She realized that although the quality of nursing care was the root of her displeasure, it was not the focus of her immediate concern. She framed her initial problem as, "Can I continue to function as director of OT if there is no change in the quality of nursing care?" She quickly went through the problem-solving process and determined that she could not accept the status quo in nursing care.

Ms. Bryant then phrased the next problem as, "Do I resign from RRC or will I stay and continue to fight?" Once again she carried the problem-solving process through to completion and determined that because of her and her staff's concerns for patients she would not resign. Her next thought was, "Now that I have decided to stay and fight, what do I do next?"

After a period of deliberation, Ms. Bryant developed the following problem statement. "Given the recalcitrance of the director of nursing and the director of rehabilitation services to respond favorably to requests for improved nursing care, what strategies might be developed and implemented to effect a positive change?"

Having progressed to Step 3 (Investigating), Ms. Bryant concentrated on the types of information she would need. Among the major questions were the following:

1. Which persons have contributed directly or indirectly to the inadequate level of nursing care and the stalemate relative to correcting the situation?
2. What acts of omission or commission are attributable to each of the persons identified above?
3. Who may be allies in the struggle to improve nursing care?
4. What information pertaining to those allies would be helpful?

Respond to Ms. Bryant's questions before reading further.

Ms. Bryant responded to her questions in the following way:

1. Contributors to the Problem

Directly	Isabel Hurley, director of nursing Nursing supervisors Nursing staff Tom Bacon, director of rehabilitation services
Indirectly	Dr. Earley, medical director James Sharpe, vice president for patient care Medical staff Patient representative Performance Improvement Committee

2. Acts of Omission and Commission

a. Director of nursing, Isabel Hurley—Relegates positioning, PROM, and ADL to low-priority status. Refuses to support OT in providing these services and denies director of OT the opportunity to meet with her and supervisors.
b. Nursing supervisors—Unwilling to demand more of the nursing staff, seemingly content with status quo.
c. Nursing staff—Unwilling to provide regular prescribed care with regard to positioning, PROM, and ADL.

d. Director of rehabilitation, Tom Bacon—Failed as an advocate for OT and was ineffective in negotiating a change in nursing attitudes and behavior. His bureaucratic behavior stifled OT director.
e. Medical director, Dr. Earley—Conspicuous in his absence of involvement in the issue of nursing care. Made no demands on Nursing to upgrade its service and comply with patient care as prescribed.
f. Medical staff—No evidence of awareness or concern about the status of nursing care.
g. Performance Improvement Committee (includes Hurley, Bacon, Earley, and three staff nurses)—Took no action against Nursing based on OT's concerns.
h. Patient representative—Either was not approached by patients, or was ineffective.
i. Vice president for patient care, James Sharpe—Contributed to nursing understaffing?

3. Potential Allies

Medical director
Medical staff
Patient representative
PT director/staff
Speech director/staff

4. Information Regarding Potential Allies

Medical director	a. Is he aware of the situation? b. If aware, is he concerned? c. Is he willing to do something to effect change?
Medical staff PT director/staff Speech director/staff	a. Are they aware of the situation? b. If aware, are they concerned? c. Have they tried to effect change in the past? If so, what happened?
Patient representative	a. Has she received any complaints about nursing service from patients or patients' families? b. If so, what were her actions and what were the results of those actions? c. If she has not received any complaints, is she aware of the situation? d. Is she willing to work with others to effect change?

Ms. Bryant realized that it would be virtually impossible to gather all the information required without assistance. A solo effort would be excessively time consuming and likely to be detected and squelched. She recruited the assistance of her own staff and the director of PT. Between them they identified strong professional or personal relationships existing between staff and the individuals about whom they wanted information. For example, one of the OTs commuted and was friendly with the patient representative. One of the PTs had a very positive working relationship with one member of the medical staff. Other relationships offering the possibility of frankness and confidentiality were noted and tapped. Within a week or so, most of the information desired flowed in as fact or reasonable conclusion. Ms. Bryant then gathered the assembled information and organized it, with the following results:

Dr. Earley, medical director, has had a lengthy professional relationship with Ms. Hurley and has respect for her as a nurse and administrator. He has been aware of shortcomings in nursing care as perceived by Ms. Bryant and has discussed them with Ms. Hurley privately. Ms. Hurley defended her service on the basis of a shortage of nursing staff and an inability to expand the staff because of a combination of inadequate funding and difficulty in recruiting when vacancies occur. Dr. Earley has accepted this explanation, therefore, he has consistently overlooked nursing deficiencies while functioning as a member of the Performance Improvement Committee. Furthermore, although he was in an excellent position, medically and administratively, to forcefully request increased funding for Nursing, he did not do so. His noncritical attitude seems to have influenced Mr. Bacon who assumed "If things are acceptable to Dr. Earley, they are acceptable to me." As a result, Nursing did not receive the criticism it merited at performance-improvement meetings.

Most of the medical staff recognized the deficiencies in nursing service and (1) complained directly to nurses with only short-lived improvement at best and (2) complained to Dr. Earley who inevitably responded that he would talk with Ms. Hurley. Those physicians who had been on staff for many years learned that their complaints to Dr. Earley were a waste of time. From time to time they exploded at nursing staff in frustration. Several expressed a genuine concern about the situation and expressed a willingness to collaborate with other services to actively bring about desired change.

The patient representative received no formal complaints about the quality of nursing care from either patients or their families. She admitted that she had long harbored a suspicion about nursing deficiencies but was of the opinion that the initiative for remediation rested with medical and rehabilitation staff. She did express concern about the patients' welfare and indicated a willingness to use her position to support appropriate efforts to improve patient treatment.

One other important piece of information gathered by Ms. Bryant related to the staff/patient ratio in Nursing. On the basis of patient population, staffing barely met minimal acceptable standards. Furthermore, there was history of delay in filling vacant positions, suggesting that Ms. Hurley's defense of Nursing was somewhat justified.

Reflecting on this additional information, Ms. Bryant reviewed and confirmed her problem statement.

What strategies might be developed to effect a positive change? Consider the positive and negative factors associated with each.

SCENARIO: CASE 18

PLEASE SAY "I DON'T KNOW"
Independence Versus Interdependence

Upstate Home Health Agency is a comprehensive and progressive home-care organization serving a geographic area roughly 30 by 40 miles, encompassing Sagamore, a city of slightly more than 100,000. The agency is part of a large integrated health system. One of the outstanding characteristics of the organization has been the excellence of its leadership, from the top corporate management through its component agencies and service departments.

One of UHHA's top managers is Sue Finnegan, PT, Director of Physical Therapy. She joined UHHA 7 years ago when she was appointed director following a 15-year career in which she worked in a variety of settings and held several administrative positions. Within the organization and among her peers she is highly respected as an effective PT and administrator. The growth and quality of PT service is credited to Ms. Finnegan, and she enjoys the loyalty of her staff. The PT operation, which is characterized by the quality of service provided and the strong morale of its members, is respected and appreciated as being well organized and efficient.

Ms. Finnegan, upon joining UHHA, quickly came to appreciate that physical therapy in a home setting is quite different from physical therapy in an institutional setting. Whereas the institutional PT functions within a defined physical parameter and is almost always within close range of associates and supervisor, the home health PT practices independently in a wide geographical area, in many different types of homes. The opportunity for direct and indirect supervision within most institutional settings is readily available, which is not the case in home health. Ms. Finnegan recognized that the ideal home health PT, in addition to possessing professional knowledge and skills, must be endowed with the qualities of confidence and maturity and with the ability to function independently and to recognize and admit limitations. For this reason she followed a policy of hiring experienced PTs whenever possible. That policy was evidenced by the fact that her staff included a number of part-time, but experienced, individuals.

Recently, however, because of the departure of one of her PTs and the ever-increasing demand for PT services, Ms. Finnegan found it necessary to employ full-time a new graduate of the State University's School of Physical Therapy. She and her supervisors had singled out Bill Talbott from all the other inexperienced applicants for several reasons. He was highly praised by the school's academic faculty and highly recommended by the clinical faculty who observed him in his clinical education affiliations. Mr. Talbott, at 27 years of age, was older than many new graduates. Before studying PT at the university, he served with distinction as a medical corpsman in the Army, including a stint in Desert Storm, the war with Iraq. He was mature, confident, and bright, and he certainly had more life experiences than most new graduates. He indicated he wanted to work in the area because his financée worked and lived in Sagamore. He preferred to work in home health because he enjoyed responsibility and the opportunity to work with a greater degree of independence.

Mr. Talbott began his orientation to the UHHA under the wing of George Breen, PT, one of the PT supervisors. The orientation encompassed all agency and departmental policies and procedures, including how to request consultation and assistance when needed. Mr. Breen took Mr. Talbott with him for a number of home visits to demonstrate the normal protocol and help Mr. Talbott get a "feel" for the area and the agency's clientele. Mr. Breen then had Mr. Talbott review a number of charts and introduced him to those patients before turning them over to him. Finally, Mr. Breen began to assign new referrals to Mr Talbott, gradually building his caseload to the expected level.

It was easy to be impressed by Mr. Talbott. He was eager, energetic, efficient, articulate, and very independent. Initial reports from his patients indicated that they liked him and had confidence in him. It was while he was digesting this wealth of positive information about Mr. Talbott that Mr. Breen was suddenly struck by a disturbing thought. Mr. Talbott had been carrying a full caseload for about a month and there had not been a single occasion in which he had requested consultation or assistance. Mr. Breen checked with the other supervisors and some of the more experienced PTs and learned that none of them had been approached by Mr. Talbott. Mr. Breen considered that to be not only rare, but unheard of!

Mr. Breen, being a conscientious supervisor, decided to look more closely at Mr. Talbott's performance. He read a number of charts of patients being served by Mr. Talbott and noted a number of questionable entries. He talked with Mr. Talbott about his caseload and interjected a number of specific questions relating to those he had when reading the charts. Mr. Talbott had a ready and confident response for each question. Unfortunately, not all the responses were appropriate! Mr. Breen relayed his actions and concerns to Ms. Finnegan. They agreed that Mr. Breen should monitor Mr. Talbott's performance more closely.

In the week following the discussion between the director and supervisor, a referral came to the agency with a seldom-seen diagnosis and one that often presents bizarre physical symptoms. Mr. Breen decided that this might be a good test for Mr. Talbott and assigned the patient, Mr. Hill, to him. Mr. Breen asked Mr. Talbott if he was familiar with the condition. When Mr. Talbott responded affirmatively, he deliberately did not test him any further. As he awaited Mr. Talbott's evaluation report on Mr. Hill, Mr. Breen called the hospital from which Mr. Hill was referred and talked at length to the PT who treated him. Mr. Breen was particularly interested in the wide variety of symptoms demonstrated and in getting a clear picture of the patient's status at the time of transfer from hospital to home.

Efficient as always, Mr. Talbott visited Mr. Hill the day after he had been assigned to him, completed all the chart work related to his evaluation the very next morning, and filed it before leaving the office to meet his schedule of that day. Mr. Breen read the evaluation report and carefully reviewed the data about symptoms and status. To his dismay Mr. Breen found a number of omissions and inconsistencies in Mr. Talbott's report. Later in the day when Mr. Talbott returned to the office, Mr. Breen asked him about his failure to note a number of specific items that had existed at the time of discharge from the hospital. Without any hesitation Mr. Talbott confidently responded by stating that those symptoms had not been present and either the hospital PT was incorrect or the patient's condition had changed.

On Friday of that week Mr. Breen asked Mr. Talbott if he had any objections to his accompanying him on a number of home visits Monday morning. Mr. Breen reminded Mr. Talbott that periodic direct observation was the responsibility of each supervisor and he had not been in the field with Mr. Talbott since the initial orientation and introduction of his first patients. Mr. Talbott voiced no objection and on Monday morning the two of them visited Mr. Hill and three other patients. While they were with Mr. Hill, Mr. Breen did some testing for those symptoms reported by the hospital PT but not by Mr. Talbott. During the other three visits Mr. Breen observed Mr. Talbott's performance very closely and listened attentively to all verbal interaction between Mr. Talbott and the patients and the patients' families. As they drove back to the office after the last visit, Mr. Breen subtly questioned Mr. Talbott about a number of issues regarding the four patients.

Almost immediately upon his return to the office Mr. Breen closeted himself in his office and recorded his observations from the morning. Among the observations were the following:

1. Mr. Hill—Several symptoms, as reported by the hospital PT, were demonstrated to be present. Mr. Talbott positively stated they had not been present the previous week and that they must have recurred.
2. Patient 2—The patient asked a question, the answer to which it was impossible for Mr. Talbott to know; nevertheless he responded as though he knew with certainty.
3. Patient 3—I asked Mr. Talbott if he was familiar with Dr. Johnson's (the referring physician's) preferred regimen for the condition being treated. He responded in the affirmative even though he had not followed that regimen with the patient.
4. Patient 4—A family member asked if the patient would achieve independent functional status, and despite the fact that it was too early to hazard an opinion, Mr. Talbott did respond in a very authoritative manner.

Mr. Breen was disturbed as he reviewed his notes relating to Mr. Talbott. He was concerned about the quality of care being provided to his patients, with particular concern for the safety of some of them. He was also concerned about the potential legal ramifications of Mr. Talbott's behavior and the reputation of UHHA. Mr. Breen relayed his observations and concerns to Ms. Finnegan. The two concluded that Mr. Talbott seemed compelled to provide an authoritative answer for everything, whether or not he truly knew the correct answer. He also seemed unable to admit he had made any error of omission or commission.

It was decided, therefore, that Mr. Breen would have a frank discussion with Mr. Talbott to inform him of their concerns and to stress the fact that no individual has all the answers all the time, nor is the best of therapists immune from occasional errors. Mr. Breen met with Mr. Talbott the next morning. Mr. Breen came away from that session with a troubled feeling. There was no counterargument from Mr. Talbott, but there was no admission of guilt either. Mr. Breen decided he was going to keep a close eye on Mr. Talbott.

As the next month passed, Mr. Breen noted that Mr. Talbott was very popular with his patients and generally performed at a more than adequate level. There were, however, a number of episodes of Mr. Talbott's missing key items when evaluating new patients or initiating questionable treatment regimens. He continued to have an answer for everything. Mr. Breen once again addressed these concerns to Mr. Talbott and emphatically stated that he must recognize his limitations and the need for assistance on occasion. Ms. Finnegan, in the meantime, was mindful that Mr. Talbott was halfway through his probationary period and reminded Mr. Breen of this fact. She indicated that she did not want Mr. Talbott to pass through probation unless they were confident that he measured up to their standards. They clearly appreciated Mr. Talbott's talents and independence, but they were nervous about "too much independence and too little humility."

Two weeks later Mr. Breen became aware of another incident of serious proportion. The situation involved a lack of knowledge on Mr. Talbott's part and resulted in his initiating a treatment regimen that was not only inappropriate, but potentially harmful to the patient. Mr. Breen immediately communicated this development to Ms. Finnegan and they agreed that they had a serious problem and something had to be done (Step 1—Recognizing).

Ms. Finnegan and Mr. Breen then stated their problem: "Mr. Talbott unnecessarily places some of his patients and UHHA in jeopardy because of his failure to admit his limitations." (Step 2—Defining.) They identified and gathered the information they considered relevant, including (1) documentation of incorrect decisions and failure to admit ignorance; (2) additional information about Mr. Talbott including his attitudes, past behavior, and overall performance; (3) his own perception and explanation of his alleged inappropriate behavior; (4) policies and procedures pertaining to the disposition of a probationary professional employee; and (5) the needs of the PT service (Step 3—Investigating).

They analyzed the information, which suggested that Mr. Talbott was a very energetic and an often innovative PT but had the potential to be dangerous to patients and the organization. The information also hinted that he might be hiding an underlying sense of insecurity and overcompensating by not admitting his shortcomings (Step 4—Analyzing). At this point Ms. Finnegan and Mr. Breen confirmed the original problem statement and prepared to move to the next steps (Step 5—Confirming).

Develop the alternatives available to Ms. Finnegan and identify and weigh the positive and negative factors associated with each alternative.

SCENARIO: CASE 19

ALLOCATION OF LIMITED FISCAL RESOURCES
Prioritization of Need

Two months ago Ms. Alice Adams, CCC-SLP/A, was appointed director of speech and audiology at Weepingwood Regional Rehabilitation Center. During the application and interview process Ms. Adams, through direct observation and information from other sources, concluded that the quality of the service provided by the department was less than it should be. Nevertheless, she accepted the position and the challenges that faced her. Administration promised support for efforts to improve the department. After 2 months on the job, Ms. Adams is now painfully aware that the situation is worse than she had originally anticipated.

During her brief term as director, Ms. Adams specifically documented her observations, analyzed them, and concluded the following:

1. The Speech and Audiology Department, to the dismay of the administration, has operated at a breakeven level for the past several years—neither generating an appreciable profit, nor incurring any significant losses. This condition prevails despite the fact that the hospital functions at, or near, full bed occupancy. Administration expects a reasonable profit from the department.
2. The staff, which includes five speech pathologists, two audiologists, and three support personnel, is perceived as conscientious but not very contemporary in their diagnostic and treatment protocols. The professional staff have not attended continuing education courses in recent years, apparently because of lack of financial support and personal apathy.
3. Much of the department's equipment is old, if not obsolete. As an example, despite a representative caseload of patients with voice and hearing difficulties, the department does not possess any up-to-date equipment for diagnosing voice or hearing dysfunctions.
4. The salary range is not competitive. Ms. Adams canvassed facilities and monitored salaries advertised in her region. Her department's salary scale is 10 percent below the median for other departments in her immediate area, and approximately 15 percent below those in the larger region in which it must compete.
5. Space is adequate for the present and the near future and would allow for a modest expansion of services.

She summarized the major deficiencies as relatively low salaries, inadequate equipment, and out-of-date protocols. She noted that the three deficiencies were interrelated. She reasoned that without higher salaries to help encourage existing staff and recruit qualified personnel, a sound continuing education plan to upgrade knowledge and skill, or the procurement of sophisticated equipment, neither the quality nor quantity of service was likely to improve.

Before submitting a proposal for administrative support to upgrade the department, Ms. Adams estimated the cost of (1) raising salaries to a competitive level, (2) purchasing modern equipment, and (3) implementing a comprehensive staff development plan. The estimates are listed below.

1. Salary increments (15% + fringe benefits) for 5 speech pathologists, 2 audiologists, and 3 support staff	$80,000
2. Diagnostic and treatment equipment	$80,000
3. Staff development (first year), including continuing education courses and professional conferences	$20,000
Total	$180,000

Ms. Adams developed a detailed report concerning departmental status and needs, including a specific budget. She presented this report to Mr. Bainbridge, the center administrator, in the form of a one-time budget request of $180,000 to supplement the regular operating budget.

One week later Mr. Bainbridge met with Ms. Adams to discuss the request. He complimented her on the quality of her report and acknowledged the validity of her stated needs. However, Mr. Bainbridge added with sincere regret, because of prior capital commitments and the center's general fiscal status, he and his board of directors had determined the maximum amount that could be made available to the Speech and Audiology Department was $100,000

Although he refrained from making a binding commitment concerning the other $80,000 requested, Mr. Bainbridge offered to make an earnest effort to provide the balance in the next fiscal year. Mr. Bainbridge indicated that Ms. Adams had full discretion in determining how to allocate the $100,000 with one caveat relating to salary increments. Because the granting of exceptional salary increments to selected employees was a highly sensitive issue, Ms. Adams would have only one opportunity to increase salaries beyond the center's routine policy. In essence, she was denied the possible strategy of providing a partial salary supplement this year with the expectation of adding the remainder the following year, if additional funds were forthcoming. Therefore, any out-of-the-ordinary salary increments must be implemented at this time or risk the possibility of no additional funds at all next year.

It is not an uncommon plight of the manager of a department to be confronted by needs that exceed available resources. In Ms. Adams' case the shortfall is $80,000, nearly half the amount necessary to implement all the proposed actions in the first year. She indeed does have a problem.

How might Ms. Adams proceed?

Step 1—Recognizing

Is there is a problem requiring action? Yes! Critical needs have been identified and, because of insufficient funds to meet all needs, those needs must be prioritized.

Step 2—Defining

Of the $100,000 pledged to the department, how much should be allocated to each of the three designated areas of need?

Step 3—Investigating

Questions

1. What are the primary needs of the department, and what is the amount needed to meet those needs?

Salary upgrade	$ 80,000
New equipment	$ 80,000
Staff development	$ 20,000
Total	$180,000

2. How much has been pledged by the administration? $100,000
3. What salary information is relevant?
   a. Currently salaries are 10 percent below other departments in the immediate geographical area, and 15 percent below comparable settings in the broader region in which the department must compete.
   b. Can a special supplement of 15 percent be divided over a 2-year period? No!
4. What are the primary equipment needs and the respective costs of each?

Videostroboscopy	$50,000
Computerized voice lab	$15,000
Soundproof audiology booth	$10,000
Visipitch	$ 5,000
Total	$80,000

5. What are the prospects for obtaining additional equipment funds in the following fiscal year? Fairly good in view of the pledge from administration.
6. Will staff be motivated to participate in professional development activities without a tangible reward? On the basis of discussions with the staff and on feedback from other reliable sources within the center, Ms. Adams concluded that most of the staff were encouraged by recent developments in the department and had a genuine desire to elevate their knowledge and skills. She also concluded that all staff felt strongly that salaries were too low.
7. What is the intensity of competition for speech and audiology personnel in the area? How critical is it for salaries to match the competition? Ms. Adams determined that, as in most parts of the country, there is a shortage of personnel in her area, resulting in about a 15 percent vacancy rate for funded positions. Although comparative information was limited, Ms. Adams concluded that the employee benefit package offered at her center was equal to,

but not superior than, benefits at competing facilities. Therefore, it seemed important for her salaries to match the prevailing rates in her area.

8. What will be the impact of a delay of at least 1 more year in the purchase of new equipment?
   a. More sophisticated diagnostic and treatment programs will be delayed.
   b. Implementation of videostroboscopy and audiology studies will not be possible for another year.
   c. The perception of the department by physicians and other referral sources will not be favorably altered.
   d. The lack of new equipment may retard staff motivation to elevate the quality of their services, particularly if there is no opportunity to employ newly learned skills.
9. If all the $100,000 is allocated to salary supplements and new equipment, will the staff take more initiative in upgrading their knowledge and skills?
   Ms. Adams concluded that the majority of the staff understood and appreciated what she was trying to do. Therefore, she anticipated there would be evidence of self-motivated professional development by at least half of the staff.

Step 4—Analysis

A thorough review of the information gathered resulted in the identification of a number of salient points:

1. The issue of salaries must be dealt with, not only for the benefit of current staff but also to enhance the department's competitive position in future recruitment.
2. If there is to be an adjustment in the salary scale, it must be accomplished at this time.
3. If the salary scale is to be adjusted the full 15 percent, there will be a shortfall of $80,000 for equipment and staff development.
4. The staff seems to be responding favorably to the new leadership in the department.
5. The prospect for additional funds for nonpersonnel items next year is relatively optimistic.
6. If the major items of needed equipment are not procured at this time there will be a delay of at least 1 year in implementing new programs.

Step 5—Confirming

The original problem is confirmed. How should the $100,000 be allocated among the three designated areas of need?

Step 6—Developing

In attempting to develop alternatives, the manager must first do some arithmetic (Tables 2 and 3).

The following six alternatives were proposed and considered by Ms. Adams.

TABLE 2
Salary Increment Options

Cost (Including Benefits)	Increment	Balance (Remaining from $100,000)
$80,000	15%	$20,000
$70,000	13.2%	$30,000
$64,000	12%	$36,000
$50,000	9.4%	$47,000
$20,000	3.8%	$80,000

TABLE 3
Equipment Purchase Options

Purchase Options	Cost	Balance Remaining from $100,000
Original request	$80,000	$20,000
Videostroboscopy only	$50,000	$50,000
Voice lab only	$15,000	$85,000
Visipitch only	$5,000	$95,000
Audiology booth only	$10,000	$90,000
Visipitch and voice lab	$20,000	$80,000
Voice lab, Audiology booth, and Visipitch	$30,000	$70,000

Although these six are not all the possible options, they provided Ms. Adams with a broad range of choices to challenge her problem-solving skills.

Alternative	Salaries	Equipment	Staff Development
1	$80,000 (15%)	$20,000 (Voice Lab and Visipitch)	0
2	$70,000 (13.2%)	$20,000 (Voice Lab and Visipitch)	$10,000
3	$70,000 (13.2%)	$30,000 (Voice Lab, Audiology Booth, and Visipitch)	0
4	$20,000 (3.77%)	$80,000 (original plan)	0
5	$50,000 (9.4%)	$50,000 (videostroboscopy)	0
6	$64,000 (12%)	$30,000 (Voice Lab, Audiology Booth, and Visipitch)	$ 6,000

Step 7—Identifying

Ms. Adams identified the following positive and negative factors associated with each alternative:

Alternative 1. This alternative brings salaries into a competitive position and provides for two of the three major items of equipment. However, it does not permit any expenditure for staff development, nor does it permit purchase of the videostroboscopy unit.

Alternative 2. Salaries are brought 3 percent above the median for the local area and within 2 percent of the median for the broader area in which the department must compete. In addition this alternative allows for the purchase of the Voice Lab and Visipitch instruments as well as providing 50 percent of the funds originally requested for staff development. As in Alternative 1 above, there are no funds for purchase of the videostroboscopy unit.

Alternative 3. This alternative increases salaries as in Alternative 2 and permits the purchase of all equipment except the videostroboscopy unit. The major advantage is raising salaries to a reasonably competitive level and obtaining some of the equipment to elevate the quality of service. The disadvantages relate to the absence of funds for staff development and the failure to purchase the videostroboscopy unit.

Alternative 4. This alternative is similar to number 2 above. Salaries are reduced by 1 percent to make $10,000 available to purchase 60 percent of the minor items of equipment originally requested.

Alternative 5. This is a radical departure from the preceding alternatives. The emphasis is on equipment, with only a minimal boost to salaries and nothing for staff development. The major advantage is the acquisition of all the equipment required to develop new programs and potentially improve the quality of service. The counterbalancing disadvantage is that salaries will continue to lag behind others in the region and there are no funds for staff development.

Alternative 6. This alternative divides the $100,000 equally between salaries and equipment. The major advantage is the acquisition of the costly videostroboscopy unit. The major disadvantages relate to no staff development funds and the inability to purchase any of the other equipment items needed. Depending on one's perspective, the salary increment of 9.4 percent may be perceived as an advantage or a disadvantage. A salary increase of 9.4 percent seems rather generous but it brings the range only to the level of the immediate local area, still 5.6 percent below the median for the broader area of competition.

Of the Alternatives, 1, 2, and 3, and even 4 to a lesser extent, may prove adequate in adjusting the salary schedule to a reasonably competitive level. In alternatives 1 and 3 staff development is completely ignored this year, and in 2 and 4 it is allotted only 50 percent of the original request. Another very serious liability to these four alternatives is that the videostroboscopy unit of choice is not affordable this year. This may perpetuate a major deficit in the evaluation and treatment of many of the patients with voice problems.

Alternatives 5 and 6, conversely, permit the purchase of the videostroboscopy unit, but sacrifice staff development and adequate salary increases.

In weighing the alternatives two critical points must be considered. Any special salary adjustment is a one-time-only proposition. Administration has emphatically stated it will not consider a special adjustment spaced over 2 years. The second critical point to remember is that the only money guaranteed to the department is the $100,000 pledged for immediate use. Despite the good faith promise to "try to satisfy the unmet needs next year," there is no assurance the extra $80,000 will be available. It is likely that most managers faced with this dilemma would favor alternatives that provide a salary increase of at least 10 percent.

Are there other alternatives to consider before proceeding to Steps 8, 9, and 10?

Steps 8–10

Weighing and Choosing Alternatives and Evaluating the Outcome

SCENARIO: CASE 20

PROMOTE FROM WITHIN OR HIRE FROM OUTSIDE?
Individual and Organizational Advancement

Three years ago Ms. Linda Brown, PT, was hired to replace the director and only physical therapist at Hope Hospital, who was relocating because of a change in her husband's employment. Prior to Ms. Brown's arrival, the PT service was characterized as adequate, conservative, and unimaginative. Ms. Brown, however, was progressive, dynamic, and innovative, and she implemented changes that resulted in a greater variety of services, a higher quality of service, and more effective marketing of services. The department grew rapidly over the 3 years.

At the present time Ms. Brown's department includes a professional staff of seven PTs, including one officially designated as assistant director, two senior PTs, four staff PTs, and support personnel. Ms. Brown delegated a number of administrative responsibilities to the assistant director, including (1) day-to-day supervision of the two senior PTs and four staff PTs and (2) direct participation with her in departmental planning and budgeting. The two senior PTs do not have major supervisory or administrative functions. They are designated as "senior" on the basis of clinical expertise and responsibility for special programs relating to industrial PT and sports PT.

Recently the assistant director submitted her resignation to accept a position as director of physical therapy at another institution. Ms. Brown took stock of her situation and decided several things:

1. There is a need for an assistant director.
2. For the present and immediate future, the duties of the position need not be changed.

3. Prior administrative experience, although preferred, is not a requirement for the position.
4. Because of both intrinsic and extrinsic factors, Ms. Brown anticipates continued growth of the hospital and her department. She expects the assistant director will have added administrative responsibilities in the not too distant future.
5. Because of the anticipated events stated in 4, Ms. Brown wants to recruit an individual with leadership potential and vision.

Ms. Brown encouraged members of her staff to apply for the position and, in accordance with the equal employment opportunity policy of the hospital, advertised in appropriate settings and professional newsletters to solicit external applications. Ms. Brown screened all the applications, including one from the senior PT responsible for the sports PT program. Ms. Brown and her staff conducted a series of interviews with the most qualified of the candidates. The outcome was that all concerned rated two individuals as the top candidates—the senior sports PT and an external candidate.

Ms. Brown then summarized the personal and professional data of the two finalists for the position of assistant director. In an effort to make a choice between the two, she listed the perceived strengths and weakness of each candidate as follows:

Internal Candidate (Senior Sports PT)

PT Experience	7 years.
Specialization	Sports PT—3 years, with certification as athletic trainer.
Administration	No formal training or experience. Has had responsibility for organizing and conducting the sports PT program in the department for the past 3 years, but her only supervisory experience relates to clinical supervision of PT assistants.
Miscellaneous	Recent work performance evaluations completed by Ms. Brown rated her as outstanding in clinical performance, responsibility, initiative, organization, and time management. She was praised as being a cooperative member of the department and one who has been popular with colleagues. There had been no indication of personal or professional character deficits that might diminish her suitability for the position of assistant director.

External Candidate

PT Experience	11 years.
Specialization	No specialty. Her entire career has been in acute-care settings similar to Hope Hospital.
Administration	In reverse chronological order, she had 3 years experience as director of a department with 10 PTs; 3 years as assistant director of a department with 20 PTs; and 3 years as a team leader.
Miscellaneous	She made a very favorable impression on Ms. Brown and the entire staff. She was very personable, and obviously a well-informed and experienced professional. She left her last position because her husband was transferred to this area. Her references from each of her three previous employers were glowing in their praise of her clinical and administrative skills. There was unanimity in praising her leadership, communication skills, planning and organizing, vision, and interpersonal attitudes and skills. When asked if she thought she could be content in the role of assistant director after having been a director for 3 years, she replied that she and her husband had discussed the matter prior to his having accepted the transfer. She had investigated the opportunities in the immediate area and learned there were no director vacancies. After much consideration she decided she could be happy as an assistant director if associated with an acknowledged leader, such as Ms. Brown, and in a dynamic and growing department such as the one at Hope Hospital.

Ms. Brown then further condensed the information about the two candidates into a succinct list of positive and negative factors, as follows:

Internal Candidate

Positive Factors	***Negative Factors***
Knowledge of department	Lack of administrative experience
Knowledge of personnel	Potential effect on sports PT
Well-liked by colleagues	
Promotion would give credence to staff perception of opportunity for upward mobility	

External Candidate

Positive Factors	*Negative Factors*
Administrative experience	Potential for staff rebellion
Strong recommendations	Potential drop in staff morale
Influx of new ideas	Possible resignation of the sports PT

At this point Ms. Brown is on the verge of making a choice. Do you have sufficient information to make a choice? Who would you select? Why?

SCENARIO: CASE 21

THE UNWANTED ASSIGNMENT
Incongruent Expectations

Spring Hill Center is a 300-bed extended-care facility. In recent months the facility's administrator has become increasingly concerned about the high rate of absenteeism and concomitant increase in the cost of workers' compensation insurance resulting from a high incidence of back injuries among personnel in the Housekeeping Department and in Dietary Services. The top administrative staff and the respective heads of Housekeeping and Dietary Services unanimously agreed that something had to be done to reduce the number of injuries. They decided to establish an ongoing, centerwide back injury prevention program for present employees and all new personnel. The facility administrator assigned responsibility for this prevention program to the Department of Physical Therapy.

Upon receiving the training assignment from the administration, Jan Barwell, PT, director of physical therapy, met with her assistant director, Judy Walinski, PT, to discuss the request. There was complete agreement that despite the added burden, the PT department should accept the assignment with enthusiasm and provide the training. After considering a number of candidates, the two agreed that Tom Jordan, PT, was best-qualified to develop the program.

Mr. Jordan, who had about 3 years experience in physical therapy, had started working at Spring Hill 3 months ago. He previously worked on an acute-care orthopedic team where he treated many patients with back injuries, and he had attended a short course on the development of a "back school." As a new member of the department he would not have PT students assigned to him for 6 months. Ms. Barwell believed that Mr. Jordan could organize the training program, conduct the initial series of sessions for all current personnel, and start monthly sessions for all new personnel within that time frame. Once the program was organized and implemented, the plan was for the training responsibility to be assigned on a rotating basis to other members of the staff. Ms. Barwell and Ms. Walinski agreed that Mr. Jordan should be granted a mutually agreed upon amount of release time to develop the program. Additional release time equal to the number of hours spent in conducting the sessions outside regular working hours would also be necessary, since many sessions would have to be conducted at night to cover all the different work shifts involved.

Ms. Walinski met with Mr. Jordan and thoroughly explained the request from the administration, the reasons for the request, and the agreement by the department to accept the responsibility. She explained why he had been selected to organize and initially conduct the program. She also described the plan for release time and openly discussed the odd hours in which many of the sessions would need to be scheduled. Mr. Jordan dutifully listened to Ms. Walinski, and when she finished, he politely, but firmly, stated that he did not want to develop the training program or conduct the initial sessions. He gave the following reasons for declining:

1. Lack of interest.
2. Having a greater interest in acquiring knowledge and skill related to his new job responsibilities.
3. The gross inconvenience of the anticipated schedule.
4. The proposed activity was not in his job description.

Ms. Walinski tried her best to convince Mr. Jordan that he was the logical choice by qualification and workload to meet this responsibility. Despite her effort she was unable to persuade Mr. Jordan, and he adamantly refused to accept the assignment. Ms. Walinski, disappointed and frustrated, then arranged to meet with Ms. Barwell to report on her conversation with Mr. Jordan. Upon learning of Mr. Jordan's stance, Ms. Barwell was incensed at his refusal to accept the assignment.

Ms. Barwell went to the personnel file, extracted Mr. Jordan's job description, and reviewed it carefully. She found nothing specific referring to the assignment in dispute but she did note under the section pertaining to duties the all-inclusive clause that appeared in all job descriptions which read, "and any other activity assigned by the immediate supervisor or the director." Ms. Barwell, therefore, instructed Ms. Walinski to relay this information to Mr. Jordan and to tell him that in accordance with the job description, he is officially assigned the activity of organizing and conducting training sessions in lifting techniques and back injury prevention for personnel from Housekeeping and Dietary Services. She concluded by saying, "Tell him to do it or else." Ms. Walinski relayed the directive to Mr. Jordan, who was now faced with a task he did not want and with an ominous-sounding ultimatum.

Obviously, the person with a problem at this time is Mr. Jordan. He is faced with an ultimatum containing two choices, neither of which appeals to him. Shortly before the problem befell Mr. Jordan, it was Ms. Barwell who seemingly had a problem, related of course, but different in nature. She did not take the time to go through the recommended problem-solving process. Instead she simply referred to a catchall phrase found in the duty section of most job descriptions and issued an ultimatum to Mr. Jordan.

Speculate about the potential outcomes of Ms. Barwell's action. Focus your evaluation of this case on the examination of the phrase "and any

other activity assigned by the immediate supervisor or the director," and identify and discuss the positive and negative outcomes associated with the inclusion of such phraseology in a job description.

SCENARIO: CASE 22

IS THIS COURSE NECESSARY?
A Test of Relative Values

Thomas Manor is a small subacute facility located in a suburban residential community with a high percentage of retirees. The primary role of the facility is to provide subacute care for the local community. The Occupational Therapy Department consists of the director, Ms. Kim Black, OTR/L, five occupational therapists, and several support personnel. Although the facility and the Occupational Therapy Department are small in size, the quality of service provided to clients is excellent. Because of the facility's clientele, the occupational therapy caseload is concentrated in the following areas:

1. Fractures, joint replacements, and multiple orthopedic trauma
2. Perceptual motor training
3. ADL and community re-entry skills

Ms. Black, who is in her third year as the director of occupational therapy, has a strong commitment to continuing education for her staff. This commitment is shared by hospital administration, as demonstrated by a generous allocation of funds for this purpose each year. Ms. Black's practice has been to have the therapists submit requests for the workshop(s) and/or course(s) they wish to attend in order of priority, an estimate of total cost and time from the department, and a statement of justification for each request. Ms. Black reviews the requests, approves at least one per therapist, and includes them in her departmental budget proposal. Last week Ms. Black announced to her staff that it was budget preparation time and they were to submit their continuing education requests for the coming year.

The five therapists submitted their respective requests in a timely fashion. The highest priority item for each is listed below:

Ms. Adams—Workshop on driving adaptations and highway safety

Mr. Brown—Conference on the latest developments in Alzheimer's disease

Ms. Clay—Workshop on fabrication of functional hand splints

Ms. Denny—Workshop on industrial work hardening

Ms. Eaves—College course in biochemistry (requesting tuition reimbursement and flextime to be able to attend classes and labs)

As Ms. Black reviewed the requests, she had no hesitation in approving the requests of Ms. Adams, Mr. Brown, and Ms. Clay. However, she was concerned by the priority requests submitted by Ms. Denny and Ms. Eaves. Ms. Denny, in her justification statement indicated that she had a serious interest in industrial work hardening and wanted to be involved in that area of occupational therapy in the future. Ms. Eaves, to justify her request, wrote that she had plans to become a physician and that she was advised to take a course in biochemistry before taking the MCAT (Medical College Aptitude Test). She believed this would enhance her application to medical school.

Ms. Black had not previously received requests such as Ms. Denny's and Ms. Eaves'. Recognizing the potential precedent-setting impact of her decisions, she determined that this was not the time for a hasty, gut-level action. Consequently, Ms. Black thoroughly reviewed Ms. Denny's and Ms. Eaves' history and performance in the department. What she found confirmed the impression she had about both Ms. Denny and Ms. Eaves. They were bright, conscientious, and team-oriented, and both demonstrated high levels of knowledge, skill, and patient interaction. Every continuing education activity in the past was directly related to the primary service activities of the department and resulted in improved performance.

Ms. Black then decided to discuss the unusual continuing education requests with Ms. Denny and Ms. Eaves and arranged to meet with them individually. In each case the individuals were very open and straightforward with her. Ms. Denny informed her that her long-term goal always had been to become a specialist in industrial work hardening. She accepted her present position after graduation to gain maturity and general experience before advancing toward this ultimate goal. She acknowledged that with some additional knowledge in the area of industrial work hardening she hoped to leave her present position within 3 years to establish a private practice as an industrial consultant.

Ms. Eaves, who had been hired by Ms. Black soon after she became director, informed her that she was fascinated and challenged by her work in the head-trauma unit. For some time she had been thinking of becoming a physician to be able to play a more comprehensive role in management of patients with closed head injuries. She recently talked with the dean of admissions at the State University School of Medicine and, after reviewing her credentials, he was very encouraging. It was he who advised her to take a course in biochemistry. Ms. Eaves indicated her goal was to take the biochemistry course, save as much money as possible, and apply for admission to medical school within 2 years. To address the matter of time away from the department for course attendance, Ms. Eaves produced a plan to work every Saturday rather than the usual first and third Saturday rotation, and to reduce her lunch from 1 hour to 30 minutes.

After meeting with Ms. Denny and Ms. Eaves, Ms. Black was troubled by conflicting feelings. Neither of the activities requested was of direct relevance to her department. Although Ms. Black had consistently promoted the professional and personal development of her staff, she questioned whether she could justify approval of continuing education funds for activities that were of no direct benefit to the department and would eventually result in the resignation of two valuable therapists at a time of a severe shortage of occupational therapists. She reviewed the departmental and hospital policy manuals for guidance and was disappointed to find a lack of specificity relevant to cases such as these.

Ms. Black consulted the facility administrator, who responded as follows: (1) She believed continuing education should be for the purpose of maintaining and/or improving the quality of service. (2) Therefore, she would not be inclined to endorse such requests. (3) However, since the facility policy does not expressly prohibit support of such requests and since there is the possibility of extenuating circumstances, she deferred to the discretion of Ms. Black and promised to support her decision.

Despite all her efforts thus far, Ms. Black felt she was no closer to a decision than when she first encountered the dilemma, and as she returned to her office she mused, "What should I do?"

What should Ms. Black do? Weigh the alternatives and choose for Ms. Black. Justify your decision.

SCENARIO: CASE 23

ONLY A MATTER OF TIME
Conflicting Values

Worthington Center is a 450-bed state residential facility for mentally ill and disabled individuals, located in a relatively affluent and rapidly growing area. Until about 15 years ago the area had been largely rural and sparsely populated, but then the local economy changed dramatically. A developer bought a large tract of rolling farmland and developed a residential and shopping community, complete with golf course. The area was attractive to retirees because of the mild climate and active lifestyle. Growth accelerated with the influx of younger families and older retirees seeking to escape the city. This growth was followed by the development of a large continuing-care residential facility housing 600 retirees. With the spurt in population there came the migration of more shopping facilities, service industries, and other small businesses necessary to support the growing population. Inevitable results of all this growth were gradual changes in Worthington Center from a quiet long-term care facility to a multidimensional mental health treatment center, with a variety of short-term outpatient treatment programs and substance-abuse rehabilitation and community re-entry programs.

Janet Cobb, OTR/L, arrived at Worthington Center 6 months ago, having come from a much larger medical facility in an urban area some 400 miles distant. She graduated from the state university with an advanced degree in health administration. Prior to coming to Worthington Center, Ms. Cobb had been employed in four different facilities, none for more than 3 years, with higher-ranking positions and greater administrative responsibility added at each move. She came highly recommended for the position of assistant administrator for operations, with administrative superiors and colleagues citing her organizational skills, efficiency, communications skills, and interpersonal attitudes and skill.

Now 6 months after her arrival at Worthington Center, Ms. Cobb reflected on the past half year. All things considered, she felt good about how things had gone. She was well received by Robert Adams, the center administrator, and by peers and subordinates. She liked the facility and the community and was happy to be away from the hustle and bustle of the large city. She made the transition from managing in private enterprise to managing in a state bureaucracy, with minimal frustration. She made a number of valuable contributions to each of the departments under her charge. The only negative factor that came to mind was her continued exasperation with Rosa Chung, the director of occupational therapy (OT). Although there had been no major problems with the OT Department in the past 6 months, Ms. Cobb had been constantly annoyed at Ms. Chung, who was invariably late for meetings and in submitting requests and reports. Budget requests for the coming year, for example, were to have been submitted a week ago and Ms. Chung was the only department head not to have met that deadline. Ms. Cobb still had not received Ms. Chung's request.

Ms. Chung has been at Worthington Center for 16 years. She was the only OT when she first came to Worthington Center and has served as director of OT the entire time. She has many friends throughout the facility because of her friendly manner and her long tenure. Physicians like and respect her because of her clinical skill and her positive attitude toward patient care. She is popular with her staff, although they do get annoyed with her occasionally because of administrative snafus and oversights. Ms. Chung allocates 50 percent of her time to direct patient care, despite the continuing expansion of the department and mounting administrative responsibility. She loves to work with patients and feels she leads best by example. Ms. Chung derives her greatest pleasure from demonstrating and teaching evaluation and treatment skills. In fact she often goes out of her way to coach OT students and inexperienced staff members as they work with patients.

The OT Department presently consists of 11 OTs and a variety of support personnel. The department is divided into three teams: (1) residential activities, (2) work re-education, and (3) community living skills.

The prevailing opinion is that the department is adequately staffed and the pay scale and fringe benefits are reasonably competitive. However, much of the equipment and work facilities are old and outdated, and the performance-improvement program as currently implemented is marginal at best.

As Ms. Cobb prepared to call Ms. Chung to remind her once again about submitting her budget request, she wondered whether her dissatisfaction resulted from the incongruence of their work styles or whether there was a serious problem that must be confronted. She replaced the phone, got out pad and pencil, and began to jot down her concerns. Within minutes the page contained the following entries:

1. Final copy of proposed budget is more than a week late. The original submission was flawed by errors and omissions and was not presented in compliance with the new budget format.
2. Departmental objectives were submitted late, and many of the objectives were inadequate because they were not measurable.

3. Ms. Chung almost always arrives late for scheduled meetings.
4. The department's formal Work Performance Evaluations are not up to date.
5. The required quarterly reports have been late, and they are not as informationally complete as desired.
6. There have been many unnecessary crises relating to staff continuing education. On several occasions documents for authorization of expenses were submitted at the last minute or with no prior authorization.
7. Although the members of her staff genuinely like Ms. Chung, a number of them seem irked by her frequent inaccessibility because "she is so busy."

Ms. Cobb considered the list of complaints and realized that she would never tolerate such performance from a new employee. She wondered why she tolerated it in this case. Ms. Cobb acknowledge that her patience to this point was most likely influenced by the fact that she was a relative newcomer and Ms. Chung had been at Worthington Center for 16 years and was very popular among the hospital's physicians. She admitted to herself that she could not continue to tolerate this aberrant administrative behavior. She recognized that she had a problem.

Despite the fact that she was aware of a problem relating to intolerable administrative deficits on the part of Ms. Chung, Ms. Cobb did not find it easy to clearly define the problem.

How would you state the problem?

Ms. Cobb's thoughts ran the gamut from "How to fire Ms. Chung" to "What can I do to help Ms. Chung overcome her deficits?" Because of Ms. Chung's loyalty and tenure, Ms. Cobb quickly rejected starting with the premise that Ms. Chung should be discharged. She reiterated her own unwillingness to tolerate Ms. Chung's pattern of administrative performance and a desire to remedy the situation in a positive manner. She then proceeded to define her perceived problem. "Given my assessment that Ms. Chung's administrative performance is unacceptable, what action(s) can I take to remedy the situation?"

Ms. Cobb progressed through the sequence of problem-solving steps and arrived at the point of developing a number of alternatives, including:

1. Do nothing and hope she changes.
2. Coach and supervise her more closely.
3. Fire her.
4. Demote her.
5. Place her on probation.
6. Encourage her to attend management courses.

Ms. Cobb reviewed the six alternatives. She was not happy for a number of reasons. She believed doing nothing would not result in any change of behavior. Because of her relative youth and newness Ms. Cobb was skeptical of the probability of success of the second alternative. She believed Ms. Chung was a valued and loyal employee and therefore was reluctant to opt for alternatives 3 and 4. She questioned whether probation would result in permanent changes, and although there was merit to the last alternative, Ms. Cobb was of the belief that Ms. Chung's deficits related to practice rather than knowledge. As she struggled with the list of alternatives, two other considerations intruded themselves into her thoughts. The first suggested she was reluctant to implement certain alternatives because of her newness to the situation and Ms. Chung's tenure and popularity. The second was the question of whether she was "making a mountain out of a molehill." These concerns caused Ms. Cobb to mentally back up a bit and ask herself the following questions:

1. Is Ms. Chung truly administratively inept or are there other factors to explain her many administrative shortcomings?
2. In consideration of my newcomer status at Worthington Center and Ms. Chung's status resulting from tenure and popularity, how can my perception of her administrative performance acquire credibility?

Ms. Cobb determined that employing an external consultant would be the fairest and most convincing way to arrive at answers to these two questions. She made some inquiries about qualified parties and the rates for such service. Armed with that information she met with Mr. Adams to discuss her problem. She clearly indicated how she intended to use the consultant, and asked for his authorization to proceed. Mr. Adams complimented her on her approach and gave his stamp of approval.

Ms. Cobb then had a civil but very frank discussion with Ms. Chung in which she expressed her concerns and explained her intention to employ a consultant to verify or refute her allegations and, if verified, offer suggestions to resolve the problem. Ms. Cobb presented a short list of candidates for the assignment and gave Ms. Chung the opportunity to veto any whom she thought might demonstrate a negative bias toward her.

Final arrangements were completed and a week later Professor Doris Black, an occupational therapy management expert at the state university, arrived on the scene. Dr. Black interviewed many individuals, including Ms. Cobb, Ms. Chung, members of the OT Department, physicians, and other personnel. In addition Dr. Black reviewed administrative documents and observed the activities of the OT Department. Before departing on the second day, Dr. Black met with Ms. Cobb and Mr. Adams and presented a brief oral report, with a more detailed written report to follow within the week. The detailed written report arrived on schedule, the gist of which is listed in Figure 4.

Upon reading the report, Ms. Cobb was gratified at having her assessment of Ms. Chung's performance verified. She was relieved and pleased with the recommendation, which she considered reasonable and which she hoped would be acceptable to Ms. Chung. Ms. Cobb was particularly pleased that the recommendation did not seem to involve any "loss of face" for either party. In an optimistic mood Ms. Cobb distributed copies of the report to Mr. Adams and Ms. Chung, indicating to the latter that they would meet the following week to discuss the report and a response.

The next week Ms. Cobb walked into Ms. Chung's office, cheerful and optimistic about the outcome of the meeting and the resolution of her problem. She was greeted politely by Ms. Chung, whose demeanor was neither cheerful nor optimistic. Ms. Cobb asked Ms. Chung about her reaction to the report and its recommendation. Ms. Chung replied that she thought the assessment of her performance was fair and reasonably accurate and she had no reason to dispute it. She understood the rationale

REPORT OF ADMINISTRATIVE CONSULTANT

Worthington Center
Department of Occupational Therapy

MAJOR FINDINGS

1. Occupational Therapy Department
   a. Adequately staffed
   b. Salary/fringe compensation competitive
   c. Acceptable organizational structure
   d. Quality of service, though not exceptional, is quite good
   e. Major equipment inadequate/some outdated

2. The Director of Occupational Therapy
   a. Very conscientious
   b. Very loyal to the organization
   c. Knowledgeable of administrative procedures and methods
   d. Appears "disorganized"; always seems to be in a hurry
   e. Carries a 50% caseload
   f. Very approachable but often inaccessible
   g. Very patient oriented; "loves direct patient care"
   h. Outstanding clinical teacher; enjoys teaching/demonstrating; spends much time with OT students and young staff
   i. Physicians like and respect her
   j. The administrative demands placed on her by the Assistant Administrator for Operations are fair, reasonable, and consistent with the respective positions

RECOMMENDATIONS

The Director of Occupational Therapy, in recognition of the ever-growing administrative demands of her position, should limit her clinical service and teaching to a maximum of 25% of her time. If she is unwilling or unable to do so she should be replaced.

Doris Black

Doris Black, PhD, OTR/L

FIGURE 4

for the recommendation; however, she was having a difficult time accepting it for the very reasons cited in the assessment.

Ms. Chung reaffirmed her love of direct patient care and her enthusiasm and pleasure in clinical teaching. She frankly wondered if she could be happy with only a 25 percent commitment to clinical service and teaching. Ms. Chung admitted she had thought of resigning and seeking a position that allowed for more time for patient care and teaching. However, she hated to leave Worthington Center, her friends in the facility and community, and the home she had built just a few years ago. She concluded by saying that she recognized that something had to be done, but she was not at the point where she could decide between complying with the recommendation or resigning.

This response caught Ms. Cobb totally off guard and with a mixture of emotions. Afraid of saying something she might regret, Ms. Cobb suggested that each of them take a couple of days to think things over before meeting again for a final decision. She returned to her office and, after thinking about what had transpired, decided she still had a problem.

Evaluate Ms. Cobb's decision to utilize an external consultant. What would you recommend as her next step?

SCENARIO: CASE 24

THE WEEKEND RETREAT
Power or Influence

Random County, located in a rural southern state, has a total population of just over 150,000. Metropolis, the county seat and largest city, with a population of 100,000, is located in the geographical center of the county, about 30 miles from any other large community.

Metropolis has a number of textile mills and furniture manufacturing companies that, along with city and county government, are the major employers in the county, aside from small businesses in a number of small towns. The major industry of the county is agriculture. The population of Metropolis has increased by approximately 10,000 each of the past three decades.

Random Hospital, the major hospital in Random County, is located in Metropolis. It has increased in size steadily over the years, and since 1985 it has increased capacity from 300 to 500 beds and has added a subacute facility, a home-care service, and a wellness center. This growth brought an influx of primary care physicians, medical specialists, and other health professionals to the community. Not unlike many other acute-care general hospitals in the 1990s, this hospital has difficulty maintaining its fiscal head above water. With taxpayers demonstrating a reluctance to raise taxes to subsidize the hospital, there is mounting pressure on administration for the hospital to be innovative and cost-effective.

As might be expected, the size of the Physical Therapy Department grew parallel to the growth of the facility over the past 10 years. In 1985 the physical therapy staff consisted of three physical therapists and one aide; by 1995 it included 15 physical therapists, three physical therapist assistants, two aides, and one clerical person. Regretfully, despite the increase in staff, the department has consistently failed to meet its projected budget margin in each of the past 5 years.

The physical therapy staff might best be described as journeymen. They are fairly steady and reliable, but not highly skilled, specialized, or innovative. Physical therapy services are rather traditional, with little intrusion of the latest, more advanced treatment techniques. There are no specialized teams or programs in existence. Most of the equipment is at least 10 years old.

Staff salaries are at the median level for the geographic region; however, fringe benefits are below the current median level for comparable facilities, especially in terms of continuing education. The total continuing education budget for the department is $500.

There have been six different directors of the Physical Therapy Department since 1985. None stayed longer than 2 1/2 years. A history of the arrival and departure of these six directors follows:

Name	*Term*	*Reason for Leaving*
Ms. Adams	11/1/85–3/30/86	Resigned—frustrated with lack of administrative support
Mr. Brown	4/1/86–12/31/86	Resigned for better position
Ms. Clay	1/1/87–12/31/88	Asked to resign because of huge fiscal deficit
Mr. Drum	1/1/89–6/30/90	Fired because of management style and poor staff morale
Ms. Efird	9/1/90–12/30/92	Asked to step down because of poor fiscal management
Mr. Fox	4/1/93–9/30/95	Asked to resign because of complaints from physicians about PT service

The hospital administrator, Ms. Hall, was appointed 1 year ago and is eager to bring an end to the historical troubles in physical therapy. Following the recent resignation of Mr. Fox, Ms. Hall conducted a vigorous search for a new director of physical therapy. She appointed Tom Gray, PT, to assume command on October 1, 1995. Mr. Gray was the director of a comparably sized department in his native state of New York. His department had a reputation for rendering routine and specialized services of high quality, at a sizable financial profit. His references reported that he was "tough" but fair with his staff and that he was particularly strong in siding with management when resisting demands of the hospital labor union. Following graduation from college, he was in the U.S. Army for 8 years and was a captain at the time he left the Army to enroll in physical therapy school. He has 8 years experience as a physical therapist including 2 years as director of a small department prior to his last 2 years as director of the larger department in New York. His colleagues and supervisors regarded him as ambitious and aggressive.

Upon his arrival at Random Hospital, Mr. Gray was charged by Ms. Hall to (1) operate the Physical Therapy Department at a profit, (2) improve the quality of service, and (3) develop specialized programs. Ms. Hall indicated she did not expect overnight miracles; on the other hand, she did anticipate some positive changes in a short time.

Because of the rapid and continual turnover of directors, the staff was rather set in their ways. After all, why try to adapt to a new director when directors don't stay around long? The staff had developed two informal networks. One was composed of the "old-timers" who had been through it all. The other included the relative "newcomers" who had experienced only a part of this sad episode. These two separate groups of staff tended to eat lunch, socialize, and share information independently of each other. There was unanimity, however, in the general lack of enthusiasm about still another "new boss."

So, on October 1, 1995, Tom Gray arrived at Random Hospital to change the Physical Therapy Department from a staid, unprofitable service into an up-to-date revenue center with efficient services and a variety of specialized programs. As soon as he arrived, Mr. Gray met with his staff, informed them of his plans to revitalize the department, and indicated that he looked forward to their cooperation. Following the meeting he did a thorough survey of the department's space, equipment, and other resources. He assessed the caseload and then went to his office to review the budget and other fiscal information.

Among the items discovered in the proposed budget for the next fiscal year were the following:

1. No request for capital items (equipment)
2. No increase in continuing educational funds
3. A request for an 8 percent across-the-board salary increment for all personnel (already announced to the staff by Gray's predecessor)

After much thought, Mr. Gray called Ms. Hall and asked if it was possible to submit a revised budget in which salary increments would be based on merit and limited to a maximum of 5 percent. He indicated a desire to apply the estimated savings (approximately $24,000) to continuing education. This pleased Ms. Hall. Furthermore, he extracted a promise from her that any profit during the year could be placed in a capital equipment fund.

Mr. Gray, immediately following his conversation with Ms. Hall, typed a memo to the staff that he posted on the bulletin board. In the memo, Mr. Gray indicated the plan to downscale salary increments from 8 percent to a maximum 5 percent based on merit. Needless to say, this news drew an angry reaction from the staff. Two days later, at the first of the newly instituted weekly staff meetings, one of the "senior" physical therapists expressed objection to the revised salary plan, but Mr. Gray indicated that as director of the department it was within his authority to do so. He explained that there was no hope of turning the department around without improvement in the staff's collective and individual levels of skill and knowledge. Therefore, his decision had been made and it was final.

At that same meeting, Mr. Gray announced the initiation of a new performance-improvement program. He indicated he had an outline for such a program and appointed a performance-improvement program (PIP) team of five to implement the program and report back on progress in 1 month. When the meeting adjourned, the two informal networks talked among themselves. Both complained about the salary issue and expressed fear that the performance-improvement program was for the purpose of finding fault and minimizing the merit increments. The senior physical therapists surmised that "things might be unpleasant for a while, but the new boss probably won't be around any longer than the others."

Because of the department's many administrative challenges, Mr. Gray saw the need to appoint an assistant director to relieve him of some of the day-to-day operational responsibilities. He observed staff closely for several weeks, and decided that Ms. King, although she had only 3 years experience, had the organizational skills, initiative, and leadership qualities necessary for the job. He regretted that the more senior personnel lacked these qualities, but he insisted on promoting based on aptitude for the position. He interviewed Ms. King and confirmed his belief. At the next staff meeting he announced his decision to the surprise of most, shock of some, and great dismay of the senior therapists.

In the meantime, the performance-improvement program had been initiated, and at the conclusion of the second review session he critiqued the first two progress reports. He expressed his dissatisfaction and indicated that he felt the PIP team was "too soft" and insufficiently critical of obvious performance deficits. He admonished them to accept the professional spirit of performance improvement and to identify and discuss these deficits for the sake of learning and improving quality of care.

Despite the friction between Mr. Gray and many of the staff, there were some positive changes. Mr. Gray's promotional efforts with physicians resulted in an appreciable increase in referrals and revenue. By December, the department seemed headed for a profitable year. The physicians liked Mr. Gray and appreciated his efforts to improve the department.

Mr. Gray decided he would use some of the continuing education money to subsidize a retreat at a nearby resort hotel that had an abundance of recreational facilities. His idea was to reward staff for their efforts in turning the corner fiscally and to provide a relaxing atmosphere to discuss progress, problems, and future plans. He got permission from Ms. Hall and reserved a block of rooms at the hotel for Friday and Saturday nights 6 weeks hence. And, as per custom, Gray provided the hotel with the usual financial guarantee to reserve the rooms, cancelable until 72 hours prior to arrival. He made plans for a Friday social hour and dinner, and for meetings from 8 AM to 10 AM and 1 PM to 3 PM on Saturday. The remainder of the time was free until checkout at 1 PM on Sunday. All meals and lodging for staff and spouses were to be paid by the department. He typed the schedule and made copies for all staff. At the next staff meeting he announced his plan and distributed the schedule.

During the ensuing 5 weeks, business proceeded more or less as usual. There were weekly staff meetings and PIP team meetings and the usual unofficial network talk at lunch and on other social occasions. It was clear that a number of people resented giving up "their weekend time to attend the retreat." Nothing was said at staff meetings or to Mr. Gray directly. As the time for the retreat approached, however, this festering wound erupted. On Thursday, the day before the retreat was to begin, several senior physical therapists went to Ms. Hall, the administrator, to express their displeasure with Mr. Gray and the planned retreat. They indicated they did not want to attend because of "conflicts with personal appointments." Unknown to the senior group, a delegation of "newcomer" physical therapists went to the director of personnel and lodged a similar complaint. Although expressing understanding, both the administrator and personnel director indicated that it was up to Mr. Gray to determine whether to continue with his plans, postpone the retreat, or cancel it completely. Both called Mr. Gray to advise him of their respective conversations. Mr. Gray was stunned at the news and began to deliberate about what he should do next. He chose to follow the 10-step problem-solving model.

Step 1—Recognizing

Is there a problem requiring a decision? Definitely! The staff had gone to the hospital administrator and to the personnel director and, in effect, indicated they planned to boycott the scheduled weekend retreat.

Step 2—Defining

What is the problem? The immediate problem concerns the staff's threatened boycott of the retreat only a day prior to the scheduled event. This will result in the loss of thousands of dollars because of the expiration of the penalty-free cancellation period. Mr. Gray is faced with the necessity of deciding how to respond to the threatened boycott.

Step 3—Investigating

Although the need for Mr. Gray to make a decision was precipitated by the threat of a boycott of the retreat, historical factors contributed to the crisis and are of relevance.

The Hospital

Random Hospital, as the major hospital in the county, had experienced dramatic growth in the previous decade, with a 67 percent increase in capacity from 300 to 500 beds. It should be noted also that the administrator of the hospital is relatively new, having been appointed 1 year previously. Ms. Hall demonstrated her knowledge of and interest in the lackluster performance of the Physical Therapy Department by personally leading the search for the latest director of physical therapy and in presenting him with a twofold charge involving a profitable operation with diversity and quality.

The Physical Therapy Department

The last decade was one of turmoil for the Physical Therapy Department. In that 10-year period six directors were appointed with none leading the department more than 2 1/2 years. The last four were either discharged or asked to resign. It is evident, based on the turnover of directors and the charge given Mr. Gray by Ms. Hall, that the department did not operate at a profit despite its location in the county's major hospital.

The Physical Therapy Department grew rapidly, with a five-fold increase in the number of physical therapists and physical therapist assistants. However, the newer staff were not assimilated, and there appear to be two separate groups composed of those with greater or lesser seniority. It must be assumed that previous leadership was not effective in motivating or enabling staff to grow professionally and/or develop special treatment programs. The meager allocation of funds for staff development reflected the priorities of the previous directors and set the tone for the staff.

The regular and frequent turnover of the physical therapy directors had another effect on the staff, causing them to assume that they need not necessarily respond to the leadership efforts of a director since the director was unlikely to be around very long. This attitude of complacency is a potential obstacle to a new director's ability to effect dramatic changes.

Mr. Gray

The recently arrived director brought his own history to the Random physical therapy scene. To begin with, he was an "outsider," appointed as an external candidate from another part of the country. His military background may be of significant influence in relation to his style of management. As an officer he was accustomed to giving orders and also to taking them. Thus, the "charge" from Ms. Hall was taken seriously, and with this mandate from above, Mr. Gray expected the staff's full compliance with his directives. Mr. Gray's reputation as "tough" and his history of resisting demands of the hospital union suggest that he is less than participatory in his style of management. The perception of him as ambitious and aggressive is a clue to anticipate a clash with a staff characterized as "set in their ways."

Precipitating Events

1. **The Budget.** The proposed departmental budget submitted by Mr. Gray's predecessor failed to include a request for sorely needed equipment or an increase in continuing education funds. On the other hand, the proposed budget called for a generous 8 percent salary increment for all staff. Perhaps the most significant and troublesome point is the fact that Gray's predecessor, Mr. Fox, indiscreetly informed the staff of the salary recommendation contained within the budget proposal. This caused the staff to expect a generous raise.
2. **Budget Revision.** Mr. Gray, to his credit, courageously decided to revise the proposed budget and reduce salary increments for his staff. To his discredit, however, his communication of this decision by posting a memo on the bulletin board left much to be desired. The reduction of an anticipated salary increment is a highly sensitive and potentially inflammatory issue at best and not likely to be defused by the insensitive posting of a memo. Furthermore, Mr. Gray's failure to solicit counsel from any of the staff deprived him of the opportunity to receive support from those who might have understood his motives. Lastly, when the increment issue was raised at the next staff meeting, Mr. Gray quickly "pulled rank" and refused to discuss the matter.
3. **The Performance-Improvement Program.** Mr. Gray further alienated his staff by stating that they needed to improve their collective and individual levels of skill and knowledge. However true that statement was, it registered

as a "slap in the face" to those on the receiving end. Immediately following the implication of inadequate skill and knowledge, Mr. Gray announced the institution of a new performance-improvement program. The decision to institute the program is commendable. Performance improvement is likely to have a positive effect on quality. The timing and method of delivery of the announcement came as a bombshell and left his purpose subject to misinterpretation. He failed to "sell" his idea as an accreditation requirement as well as a benefit to staff, and he failed to solicit support from within the ranks through a series of stage-setting discussions.

4. **Appointment of Assistant Director.** A physical therapy department the size of Mr. Gray's more than likely requires the services of an assistant director. Mr. Gray demonstrated administrative acumen in recognizing the need. He made the selection on the basis of organizational skills, initiative, and leadership qualities, rather than on experience or tenure alone. Nevertheless, the arbitrary method by which he made his choice, coupled with the sudden announcement, erected one more barrier between Mr. Gray and his staff.
5. **The Retreat.** It should be apparent by this stage that Mr. Gray's style of management is a paternalistic, benevolent dictatorship. His decision to reward the staff with a retreat at a location of his choice and on dates of his choice supports this conclusion. Then, with no prior orientation to the idea and no input from staff, he announced his plan and distributed his schedule of events. It is hardly surprising that antagonism toward Mr. Gray and his plan manifested itself with the "revolt."

Step 4—Analyzing

Many conclusions can be drawn from the wealth of relevant information available. The more salient conclusions are listed below:

1. The PT Department has a 10-year history of managerial turnover and professional stagnation.
2. The staff suffers from a lack of professional motivation.
3. Mr. Gray enters the scene perceived by staff as an "outsider" and just one more of a long line of interim directors.
4. Mr. Gray is highly motivated and enjoys the support of the hospital administrator. He is astute in determining the needs of the department, but his style of management in relation to decision making and communication alienates his staff.
5. The physical therapy staff, having had weeks to confront Mr. Gray with their objections to the retreat, demonstrated petty and unprofessional behavior by (a) waiting until the last day to express those concerns and (b) bypassing Mr. Gray in lodging their complaints and threatened boycott.
6. Timing is a critical factor in this dilemma. It is too late for Mr. Gray to postpone or delay the retreat without severe financial penalty. He has only hours in which to make a decision about how to proceed at this juncture.

Step 5—Confirming

The problem as initially perceived still exists: The staff has threatened to boycott the weekend retreat, and at this late date Mr. Gray and his department stand to lose a large amount of money if the retreat is postponed or canceled. Perhaps a more significant set of problems relates to the management style of Mr. Gray, the attitudes of the physical therapy staff, the resolution of recent conflict, and the development of a harmonious and productive environment in the PT department.

Step 6—Developing

Listed below are five options from which Mr. Gray might choose. Although not an exhaustive list, these are among the more obvious.

1. Proceed with the retreat as planned, with attendance being mandatory except for verified illness.
2. Postpone the retreat to a later date.
3. Cancel the retreat.
4. Call an immediate staff meeting and, following an explanation and discussion as to the purpose and potential benefits of the retreat, appeal to the staff for support, and then permit the staff to vote.
5. Proceed with the retreat, with attendance optional and with assurance of no reprisal directed toward absentees.

Step 7—Identifying

The positive and negative factors associated with each alternative are listed below.

Alternative 1—Proceed as Planned, With Attendance Mandatory

Positive Factors	*Negative Factors*
The informal setting may encourage the staff to express concerns openly; a frank discussion betweem Mr. Gray and his staff may help clear the air.	Staff resentment may escalate to a new high.
As a result of frank discussion, there may be a collaborative setting of goals and priorities for the department.	One or more staff may resign.

Alternative 2—Postponement to a Later Date

Positive Factors	*Negative Factors*
Emotions may subside and result in a more productive retreat at a later date.	The money to guarantee rooms and meals will be lost.
Mr. Gray might be looked upon more favorably by staff if they perceive his action to be out of concern for their desires.	As a result of the lost deposit, Mr. Gray's standing with Ms. Hall is likely to be diminished.
	Mr. Gray will "lose face" and his power status in the hospital as well as the department will be affected adversely.
	Postponement may set a precedent for future "revolts" whenever staff become displeased.

Alternative 3—Cancel the Retreat

Positive Factors	*Negative Factors*
Mr. Gray might be looked upon more favorably by staff if they perceive his action to be out of concern for their desires.	The money to guarantee rooms and meals will be lost.
Mr. Gray may come away from the conflict with a new appreciation of the benefits of discussion and consultation with staff.	As a result of the lost deposit, Mr. Gray's standing with Ms. Hall is likely to be diminished.
	Mr. Gray will "lose face," and his power status in the hospital as well as the department will be affected adversely.
	Cancellation may set a precedent for future "revolts" when staff become displeased.
	The opportunity for collaborative planning in the near future may be lost.

Alternative 4—Staff Meeting, With Vote

Positive Factors	*Negative Factors*
The staff may perceive Mr. Gray as more sensitive to their needs and interests.	There is the potential for angry confrontation between Mr. Gray and his staff or the possibility of passive resistance by the staff, neither of which is likely to prove beneficial.
Mr. Gray has an opportunity to explain actions and appeal to the staff for understanding and support.	A negative vote by the staff may further nurture their attitude of resistance to change.
Mr. Gray may develop an appreciation of the need to be more participatory in his management style and more open and sensitive in his communication.	A negative vote may cause Mr. Gray to lose stature with his staff and possibly with Ms. Hall.
	A negative vote will result in the loss of a considerable amount of money by the department.

Alternative 5—Proceed, With Attendance Optional

Positive Factors	*Negative Factors*
Mr. Gray may be perceived as being responsive to staff concerns.	Mr. Gray runs the risk of a total boycott with the subsequent loss of money and "face."
Even partial attendance may "break the ice" and begin the process of reconciliation and greater cooperation in the future.	The chasm between the staff's two informal groups may widen if they choose differently.

Complete Steps 8, 9, and 10 (Weighing, Choosing, and Evaluating). Weigh the positive and negative factors associated with each alternative, make a choice, and evaluate that choice.

Part II

ANALYSIS AND CONCLUDING THOUGHTS

Steps 1–10

A Sample of the 10-Step Problem-Solving Process

ANALYSIS: CASE 1

TRANSITIONS IN STYLE OF MANAGEMENT

Concluding Thoughts

There are a number of lessons to be derived from this case. The situation described is not unusual or unique. The first lesson is that an abrupt change in management style, no matter in which direction, can be very disconcerting to employees. It is important for a newly appointed manager, particularly one appointed from the "outside," to diligently gather information and develop insights about the style of management and behavior of his or her predecessor before assuming the role of leadership.

A second lesson is that trust in a new leader is not imparted immediately, particularly in those environments in which trust was nonexistent previously. Furthermore, the development of trust in a new leader is much more dependent on the actions of the leader than the words employed.

Relative to the solicitation of specific information from a group that is not responsive because of the group's lack of experience, confidence, or trust, the use of anonymous multiple-choice ballots can be a very effective tool. A staff member who might be reluctant to voice an opinion at a meeting, or in a one-on-one conference with the department head, may feel secure in this anonymous opportunity to venture opinions, estimates, and preferences without fear of ridicule or retribution. This procedure has the potential for raising the level of trust and confidence among individuals and staff collectively.

Administrators rarely make choices between black and white, but usually among shades of gray. In this particular scenario, Ms. Smith identifies three major alternatives in attempting to resolve the problem as she perceived it. There is merit to each of the alternatives and none portends dire consequences. Alternative 1 stands alone in that, if employed, it eliminates Alternatives 2 and 3. On the other hand, it is quite possible to use Alternatives 2 and 3 either in isolation or in combination with the other. The final choice of the alternative(s) will depend on how the individual manager weighs the positive and negative factors of each alternative and on that individual's degree of confidence and assertiveness.

A final lesson pertains to the strategies listed in Alternative 3. It is the firm belief of the authors that many of the strategies (praise, tactful criticism, delivery of promises, and so forth) are not specific to this situation, but should be the norm in any work environment.

Steps 1–2

Recognizing and Defining a Problem

ANALYSIS: CASE 2

REGULAR STAFF VERSUS CONTRACT PERSONNEL

The definition of the problem or the decision to be made is an important second step. It largely determines the kind of information required in Step 3. Without the relevant information, problem resolution often is less than satisfactory. In this particular case, Step 2 assumes even greater importance because of the diversity of options for defining the problem. The need to focus is critical.

Before constructing the problem statement, the manager needs to consider the series of developments and complaints. The initial set of complaints, which related to stress, overwork, and quality of patient care, were understandable and readily attributable to the ongoing shortage of staff. In retrospect, Ms. Pullen believes she took the only viable option to effect a quick remedy for the problem and does not regret making that decision.

The latest set of complaints is quite different from the first. A close look at these complaints reveals that 9 of 10 complaints relate to attitudes and work habits of the contract therapists. One pertains to the salary discrepancy between contract and regular personnel. Resolving the first 9 does nothing to resolve the complaint about salary, and though salary increments often serve as temporary satisfiers, resolving the salary issue is unlikely to resolve the other 9 complaints. Therefore, the first conclusion may be that a single statement cannot effectively embrace the complete list of complaints and demands. In effect, there are at least two distinct problems.

If one segregates the salary issue, there remains 1 demand (equal treatment of contract and regular therapists) and a list of 9 complaints. Is there sufficient homogeneity among the 9 complaints to effectively develop a single problem statement to embrace the lot? The authors suggest a further subdivision into two categories. The first includes the more tangible items related to workload, policies and procedures and the salaries of the contract employees. The second includes the less tangible items of attitudes and socialization. If one follows this approach there are now three problems.

Problem 1

Are the allegations of abuse of policies, procedures, and workload true? If so, what can be done to correct the situation?

Problem 2

Are the allegations concerning the attitudes and lack of socialization true? If so,

a. Is this a significant problem?
b. What might be done to improve the situation?

Problem 3

There is a 10 percent salary difference between the contract physical therapists and the "regulars."

a. Is it possible to raise departmental salaries to the same level?
b. Is it prudent to do so?

Having clarified the problems, the manager can now proceed to Step 3 (Investigating) to gather and organize the information that will be necessary to make a decision.

Concluding Thoughts

The focus in this case has been on the definition of the problem. As stated earlier, this is always an important step. The significance in this case is the advisability of developing more than a single problem statement to better accommodate the diversity of the complaints and demands. By doing so the manager will have a clearer picture of what information needs to be sought and will be better able to organize the information effectively.

When confronted with a situation in which multiple problem statements have been developed, the manager, before proceeding with the gathering of information, may wish to examine the set of statements or questions to determine (1) the relative priorities of the problems and (2) the logical sequence for resolution. In this case, if Ms. Pullen fails to gain the cooperation of the contracting organization by requiring their assigned therapists to abide by the policies and procedures as clearly stated in the contract, she may opt to terminate the contract. If the contract is terminated, there is no need to be concerned with the attitudes and socialization of the contract therapists. On the other hand, if the contracting organization pledges adherence to policies and procedures by assigned therapists, then Mrs. Pullen can place a higher priority on the subject of salaries. Resolution of one problem often affects the priority of associated problems.

ANALYSIS: CASE 3

WHAT WENT WRONG?

Unlike most of the cases presented in this book, this case focuses on the early recognition and prevention of a problem. It provides the opportunity to (1) determine why a problem arose and (2) describe the process of effective delegation.

Most managers, in attempting to identify the contributing errors of omission and commission, cite Mr. Bassett's failure to prepare a thorough job description including the minimal job requirements and preferences (error of omission). Many managers also cite Mr. Bassett for having committed an error of commission in appointing Ms. Gray, who had no previous administrative experience, to the newly created position. The authors agree with the first contention. In this scenario a written job description would have been helpful. Before passing judgment on the second suggested error, consider the process of delegation. Not until that process is understood can the list of errors be developed thoroughly and accurately.

Delegation is a tool of the effective manager who, in effect, works through others to achieve the objectives of the organization. Delegation is much more than the mere assignment of a task. Delegation is granting to a subordinate the right to make decisions and act on behalf of the manager within the parameters determined by the manager and agreed to by both. It is critical to appreciate that the manager, although imparting responsibility and authority to an employee, is not absolved of the ultimate responsibility for the decisions and actions of that employee.

As stated earlier, management involves working through others. Delegation is one of the methods the manager may use to work through others. Delegation may be indicated for a number of specific reasons, including development and fulfillment of the employee or accommodation for the limitations of the manager. In this particular case, apparently Mr. Bassett was motivated exclusively by the latter, namely his own limitation of time.

For delegation to be successful, a number of prerequisites must be in place. First, the employee must be groomed or prepared so that he or she is able to respond effectively to the assigned task. Second, there must be mutual recognition and acceptance of the risk involved, as there is no guarantee that all delegation will be successful. And third, there must be a climate of mutual trust and confidence, with channels of communication between the manager and employee.

Once the prerequisites are in place, the manager must be clear about what he or she is delegating and why. The manager also needs a reasonable idea of the resources (money, space, equipment, personnel, and time) he or she is willing to commit. Because the manager is ultimately responsible for the outcome, he or she must consider controls or conditions to be imposed, particularly in relation to the method and frequency of communication.

The process of delegation is not complete, however, until the employee is fully informed (and accepts) the following:

1. The specific expectations and/or outcomes anticipated
2. The extent and limits of authority and decision making
3. The frequency and method(s) of communication
4. Resources available
5. The completion deadline, where applicable

To summarize the process, the manager determines **who** is to do **what** by ***when,*** and the employee determines **how** it is to be done.

So now we return to the original question, "What went wrong?" The errors of omission and commission can be identified by reviewing the prerequisites for successful delegation. There did seem to be a feeling of mutual trust and confidence between Mr. Bassett and Ms. Gray. On the surface at least, there was an openness in communication despite busy schedules and limited accessibility. On the basis of the information presented in the case study, there is no evidence that either party gave any thought to any risks that might be involved. The critical error, however, is one of omission on the part of Mr. Bassett. He completely ignored the prerequisite pertaining to grooming and preparation. Ms. Gray had no administrative experience prior to joining Mr. Bassett in his practice. There is no evidence to suggest that he attempted to prepare Ms. Gray or any of his employees for administrative tasks. Difficult as it may be to believe, Mr. Bassett did not even ask Ms. Gray if she felt capable of meeting the responsibilities thrust at her!

Mr. Bassett appeared to have a clear idea of what he was delegating and why. He was negligent, as was Ms. Gray, in failing to discuss the resources (particularly time) required to meet the delegated responsibilities. It appears as though Ms. Gray was encumbered with administrative responsibilities without a reduction in patient-care responsibilities. Another major error of omission by Mr. Bassett was the failure to install controls relating to the responsibilities delegated. He did not, for example, suggest weekly meetings to discuss progress or problems. There were no agreed-upon predetermined milestones or schedules for development of documents or for submission of preliminary drafts, and no way to let Mr. Bassett know if help was needed.

Relative to the act of delegation, Mr. Bassett committed numerous sins of omission. He failed to propose details pertaining to the method and frequency of communication, and he failed to allocate the resource of time. This might have been done by proposing to Ms. Gray that she reduce her patient-care activity by 20 percent and devote that time to her new administrative responsibilities. As it turned out, Mr. Bassett's greatest sin of omission was his failure to convey a deadline for the completion of the work-performance standards, evaluation documents, and the performance-improvement program. Had he done so, or had Ms. Gray inquired and been more informed, it is quite likely that the outcome would have been more satisfying to both parties.

Concluding Thoughts

The authors have heard many management colleagues proudly boast, "When I delegate something, I turn it over completely and keep my nose out of it." This approach to delegation is ill-advised. First, just as an athlete improves performance as the result of feedback from the coach, and as a student learns from the critique of assignments by the teacher, so is the employee likely to learn and develop confidence from the coaching and feedback of the manager during the process. Second, since the manager is ultimately responsible for the outcome, it is clearly in his or her best interest to develop controls and to establish regular patterns of communication throughout the process.

ANALYSIS: CASE 4

DECLINING WORK PERFORMANCE

Most managers quickly recognize, as did Ms. Gonzalas, the existence of a problem and acknowledge the need for a solution. Step 2 is to define the problem. In this case, defining the problem is complicated by Ms. Gonzalas's concern not only for the performance of assigned administrative duties but also for the well-being of Ms. Parsons as a friend and colleague.

For the manager whose only concern is job performance, the development of a problem statement is relatively simple. The problem may be defined as any of the following:

1. What can be done to restore Ms. Parsons' work performance to its former level?
2. Should I demote Ms. Parsons and replace her with one of her staff?
3. Should I terminate Ms. Parsons?

For those who share Ms. Gonzalas's values and philosophy, however, the existence of a concern for the individual complicates the process of problem solving. The focus is no longer on job performance with potential remedies being rejuvenation, demotion, or termination of Ms. Parsons. Now the manager's concern for the physical, mental, and financial status of Ms. Parsons must be addressed in the problem statement. Two sample statements, one positive and one negative, appear below.

1. What action(s) can be taken to (a) facilitate a more efficient and effective discharge of assigned administrative responsibilities, (b) increase Ms. Parsons' job satisfaction, (c) reduce her job-related stress, and (d) assure her fiscal stability?

2. What action(s) can be taken to facilitate a more efficient and effective discharge of assigned administrative responsibilities without physical, mental, or financial detriment to Ms. Parsons?

The manager must appreciate that Step 3 in the problem-solving process (Investigating) is influenced by the problem definition. The inclusion of the human concern will add to the number and alter the types of questions asked when seeking information necessary to resolve the problem. The manager might ask the following relevant questions:

1. Can the department continue to function at the present level of performance by Ms. Parsons? If yes, then the manager must ask, "Am I willing to accept that level of performance?
2. Is it possible to ease Ms. Parsons' workload by
   a. Reorganization?
   b. The addition of another clerical person?
   c. Streamlining operational procedures to reduce the demands of professional staff on clerical staff?
3. Will administration consider job reclassification for Ms. Parsons with no reduction in pay?
4. Will Ms. Parsons be willing to accept another position in the department at a lower classification and under the supervision of one of her present supervisees at
   a. Her present rate of pay?
   b. A reduced rate of pay?
5. Are there other positions in the hospital, at the same job classification level but of a less demanding and stressful nature, for which Ms. Parsons is qualified and from which Ms. Parsons is likely to derive greater job satisfaction?
6. Would an improvement in Ms. Parsons' computer skills add to her efficiency and reduce job stress? If so, what strategy(ies) could be employed to accomplish this?
7. Is there, in fact, an excessive amount of turnover among clerical staff in the department? If so, what is at the root of the rapid turnover, and what can be done to reduce the rate?

Concluding Thoughts

The focus of this case is the influence of the manager's values and philosophy on the definition of the problem. The character of the problem statement will determine the kind of information required to move on to decisions and ultimate problem resolution. The questions posed are not based solely on the assumption of Ms. Parsons' shortcomings but also on the possibility of shortcomings in the "system."

This case is an example of a situation where Steps 3 (Investigating) and 4 (Analyzing) may result in a major revision of the problem statement or in the severe limitation of the number of alternatives available for consideration. If, for example, Ms.

Gonzalas learns that Ms. Parsons adamantly refuses reassignment and reclassification, even at no reduction in pay, Ms. Gonzalas will be forced to revise the problem statement drastically. On the other hand, if Ms. Gonzalas learns that despite Ms. Parsons willingness to be reclassified, the hospital administration will not permit reclassification and retention of existing salary, the problem statement will remain unaltered but one potential alternative will be eliminated.

Throughout this book there are references to values and their influence on behavior and decision making. This case highlights that concept. The manager's values determine the essence of the problem definition. That definition provides the foundation for all actions toward problem resolution.

ANALYSIS: CASE 5

ROMANCE IN THE WORKPLACE

Office romances often lead to "wicked" problems for managers. The 10-step problem-solving approach applies but requires very skillful consideration at each step. Deciding when and if to intervene and predicting the response of individuals to any chosen intervention is always difficult.

Ms. Reona had a difficult time focusing. She remembered the late nights at the office and recalled that on each of those occasions Mr. Jordan and Ms. Winthrop had been working late too. Were they eagerly waiting for her to leave? She also recalled how she had found the letter from Ms. Winthrop requesting a transfer from the satellite office just sitting on her desk. At the time it had not occurred to her to wonder how it had gotten there. Had Mr. Jordan placed it there later that same night? What other signs had she missed?

Oh! And Mrs. Jordan is such a dear friend. She always believed the Jordans had a wonderful marriage. How could he do this to her? Was it true? Perhaps it was all circumstantial. Office gossip is often wrong. Why hadn't she thought to ask for more details, for proof?

Recognizing that wrestling with the problem in this emotional fashion was of no value, Mrs. Reona pulled a notepad from her purse and attempted to clarify the problem in writing. She considered the following potential problem statements.

1. Are Ms. Winthrop and Mr. Jordan having an affair?
2. How can I find out for sure?
3. If they are having an affair, is it anyone's business but their own?
4. Has this alleged affair influenced Ms. Winthrop's work performance in any negative way?
5. Other than a bit of extra chatter and whispering around the coffee pot, has this alleged affair affected office activities or patient care in any negative way?
6. Is Ms. Winthrop the victim of sexual harassment?
7. Should I tell Mr. Jordan's wife?

8. Should I tell Ms. Crowly?
9. Should I tell Mr. Jordan and/or Ms. Winthrop that their alleged affair is the hot gossip of the week?

As usual, the exercise of writing problem statements helped Ms. Reona focus on the facts and the realities of the situation. Ms. Reona accepted ownership for only two of the original problem statements she constructed. One was the dilemma as to whether or not she should tell Mr. Jordan (or Ms. Winthrop) that this alleged affair was the topic of office gossip. The second was a personal, rather than a professional, problem. As she is close friends with the Jordans, she questioned her responsibility to both husband and wife. Fortunately, personal problems are beyond the scope of this text. (Perhaps Ann Landers could help!)

The authors suggest that it is rarely in the best interest of the manager to attempt to determine the truth of such allegations. There is no indication that the alleged relationship interferes with Ms. Winthrop's work performance, and Ms. Reona is in no position to evaluate the work performance of Mr. Jordan. There is no evidence or complaint of sexual harassment. The problem of whether to tell Mr. Jordan or Ms. Winthrop, however, is a sticky one. The reactions of either are most unpredictable. The messenger in such cases is often the one who is shot! The decision about taking that risk must be based entirely on instinct and the nature of Ms. Reona's professional and personal relationship with Mr. Jordan. Even if she chooses to tell Ms. Winthrop, she can be reasonably sure the message will be relayed to Mr. Jordan. The authors suggest that the other problems identified may best be left to resolve themselves.

Concluding Thoughts

Generally, interoffice romances, regardless of their perceived propriety, are beyond the scope of the manager's interest, as long as they remain outside the office. Unfortunately, many such relationships do have an impact on office operations either through changes in work performance or, as is most likely, through the eventual resignation of one or both parties. Unacceptable changes in work performance must be handled directly and rationally, as they would be in any other circumstance. Resignations may be unavoidable.

ANALYSIS: CASE 6

THE JOKE'S ON YOU

This case is an unfortunate, but all too common, example of interpersonal relationships gone awry. Each member of Mr. Rosetti's staff interpreted his well-intended, friendly behavior differently. He was well-liked, and he believed that all his staff enjoyed his efforts at humor, even if somewhat off-color. He believed that they appreciated his reassuring and innocent physical contacts and that they were flattered by his attentiveness to their personal appearance. As the newcomer, Ms. Hopkins obviously had a different interpretation.

Depending on your own perspective about appropriate office interactions between members of different sexes, it is easy to paint either Ms. Hopkins or Mr. Rosetti as the villain in this drama. The relationships between Mr. Rosetti and the staff seemed to be fine before Ms. Hopkins arrived. Perhaps others among the staff shared similar but less potent concerns, but were more willing to be tolerant or were too fearful to admit their discomfort or displeasure. Those individuals might perceive Ms. Hopkins as the heroine with the fortitude to confront a sensitive problem. Others among the staff may resent Ms. Hopkins for disrupting a congenial and friendly office and for accusing Mr. Rosetti unjustly.

Either way, the stage is set. A complaint of this nature will be taken seriously by the personnel office regardless of the administration's previous impression of Mr. Rosetti. Formal grievance procedures will be followed, and both Ms. Hopkins and Mr. Rosetti can look forward to an emotionally charged few months. The outcome at this juncture is unpredictable.

Concluding Thoughts

The clear lesson of this case is the power of prevention. In spite of his good intentions, Mr. Rosetti was a sexual harassment case waiting to happen. In today's work environment, where issues of gender bias and sexual harassment lurk at the forefront of everybody's mind, managers cannot afford to risk physical contact or conversation that might be interpreted by any reasonable person as sexual in nature. Similar risks exist among peers, but the added element of a supervisory relationship and the power of a management position multiply that risk exponentially. Today's manager, whether male or female, must learn techniques to create a friendly office environment without risking misinterpretation or inadvertently offending members of either gender. Although the example in this case may seem frivolous, it does indeed constitute sexual harassment in many work environments. An element of coercion certainly adds to the seriousness of the offense but is not necessary for determining harassment. An action or communication that is offensive to a "reasonable individual" is sufficient.

ANALYSIS: CASE 7

WHAT ARE YOU GOING TO DO ABOUT IT?

Step 1—Recognizing

Is there a problem requiring a decision or action? Yes! Students have been scheduled for the Trauma Center for nearly a year and the new trauma team leader refuses to accept the students. The question of who owns the problem, Mr. Sawyer or Ms. Branch, is important. Mr. Sawyer must take some action, even if it is to tell Ms. Branch to handle the problem herself.

Step 2—Defining

What specific action should Mr. Sawyer take regarding the students' assignment to the Trauma Center and Mr. Jackson's refusal to accept the students? What action should Ms. Branch take?

Step 3—Investigating

Some facts are known and additional information is needed.

What Is Known

1. The clinical education assignment
   a. Affiliation with the schools is long-standing.
   b. The schools have a history of being very dependable.
   c. The students, through their faculty, specifically requested the Trauma Center.
   d. Ms. Branch arranged the assignments to the Trauma Center nearly a year ago.
   e. All other clinical instructors are committed for that time period.
   f. Students were assigned to the Trauma Center in the past.
2. Ms. Branch
   a. She is considered to be organized, efficient, effective, and fair.
   b. By title, she has been delegated administrative authority in matters relating to clinical education.
   c. She agreed to the Trauma Center assignment a year ago on the basis of existing operating policies and practice and with the approval of the trauma team leader at that time
   d. She gave Mr. Jackson 1 month advance notice about the upcoming assignments.
   e. She did not discuss clinical education for students with Mr. Jackson prior to her informing him of the assignments.
3. Mr. Jackson
   a. He has an excellent clinical reputation and has demonstrated superior performance.
   b. He had not revealed at any time his aversion to students in the Trauma Center.
   c. Officially, on matters relating to clinical education he is under the authority of Ms. Branch, center coordinator for clinical education.
   d. He had not been informed during job interviews or during orientation that he was expected to teach students in the Trauma Center.

What Is Unknown

1. Ms. Branch—What is her likely reaction if Mr. Sawyer defers to Mr. Jackson and cancels the students?
2. The schools—What is the likely reaction of the schools if the students' affiliations are canceled?
3. Mr. Jackson—What is his likely reaction if he is required to accept the students?
4. The clinical education assignment
   a. Are the other trauma center therapists willing to accept the students?
   b. Do the students still have a serious interest in trauma care?
   c. What is Mr. Jackson's likely reaction if the students are assigned to members of his staff?

As concluded from the list of questions identified in Step 3, there are factors that go far beyond logistics. Issues of major importance, such as authority, precedent, and affiliation with reliable educational institutions, override simple scheduling and individual preference. The effective manager recognizes the far-reaching implications of the problem and seeks out and considers information beyond simple scheduling concerns.

Steps 4, 5, and 6—Analyzing, Confirming, and Developing

Now analyze the information and develop alternatives for action.

The outcome of the process will be a decision resulting in a specific action to resolve the immediate dilemma. Mr. Sawyer and Ms. Branch must recognize the cause of the problem and the steps that can be taken to prevent a recurrence in the future.

Concluding Thoughts

In this case, Mr. Sawyer, as director of rehabilitation, has the authority to mandate a specific policy regarding clinical education in the Trauma Center. However, he appreciates that he has, in fact, delegated certain authorities to Ms. Branch in her role as center coordinator for clinical education and to Mr. Jackson as the lead therapist in the Trauma Center. In order to maintain the authority and the integrity of their respective administrative positions, Mr. Sawyer challenged Ms. Branch and Mr. Jackson to develop a mutually agreeable clinical education policy for the Trauma Center.

The authors commend Mr. Sawyer for not participating in the discussions and not intervening in any way. Providing the opportunity for employees in conflict to resolve problems is a useful strategy for managers. For Mr. Sawyer to issue a mandate would very likely alienate at least one, if not both, of the two supervisors. If Ms. Branch and Mr. Jackson are unable to reach agreement, Mr. Sawyer may need to provide additional structure for the negotiation process. He may need to make clear his expectation that they resolve the problem and suggest guidelines for problem solving. Requiring employees to accept responsibility for problem resolution within the scope of their authority and responsibility is important in grooming employees for future management responsibilities.

Steps 3–5

Investigating, Analyzing, and Confirming the Problem

ANALYSIS: CASE 8

HOW WILL YOU KNOW?

Much has appeared in management literature about the need for measurable organizational objectives and quality indicators. Unfortunately, whereas the leading dictionaries treat words such as objective, goal, aim, and target more or less synonymously, many management authorities do not. Some distinguish these words on the basis of major versus minor or distant versus immediate. For the purpose of this exercise the authors liken "objective" to the rose, which "by any other name would smell as sweet." The authors consider an objective something to strive for or attain, a desired state. It matters less what one labels the desired result than that it be recognized for what it is—something to strive for or at which to aim.

The authors readily commiserate with Ms. Strong and her dilemma concerning the development of objectives, yet concur readily with Ms. Yancey in her demand for measurable statements. The road to success in attempting to meet this challenge is to do so by implication. Although quality itself cannot not measured, factors and measurable criteria that contribute to or detract from quality can be assessed. One cannot measure the talent of a basketball player, but one can measure the player's height, speed, vertical jump, shooting percentage, and so forth to arrive at a reasonable conclusion. So it is with the factors Ms. Strong is asked to put into measurable terms.

An objective should not be confused with a strategy or activity, which is a means to the end. Objectives are not attained by simply being stated. Objectives must be meaningful and challenging, and they require enabling strategies to be attained. A simple example is the student whose objective is to earn an "A" in a course. A reasonable strategy is to study the course material for at least 1 hour per night. Objective and strategy are closely linked, but they are distinct entities.

Below are the five objectives of concern to Ms. Strong and Ms. Yancey. Ms. Strong provided the lettered items, which might be considered subobjectives to support the primary objective.

1. To provide high-quality speech and audiology service
   a. Client/family satisfaction—The target is an average score or rating of not less than 4 on patient exit survey forms; a log will be kept of all formal comments and correspondence indicating satisfaction or dissatisfaction. Complaints will be acted on immediately with documentation of action taken.
   b. Physician satisfaction—A record of all positive and negative comments from physicians will be maintained. All complaints will be acted on immediately with documentation of action taken. No more than three complaints will be received per year.
   c. Collective and individual performance on peer reviews—Peer review scores for all items will exceed "minimal passing."
   d. Attainment of treatment goals—Outcomes will be compared favorably with initial goals and the anticipated time frame for 80 percent of sample cases reviewed for established critical pathways.
   e. Presentation/attendance at in-service education programs—One in-service program will be presented each month with at least 70 percent of staff present. Follow-up evaluation forms will be used to assess the application of new information learned 1 month following each in-service presentation.
   f. Staff attendance at off-campus continuing education programs—Eighty percent of the staff shall attend at least one educational program external to the institution. Staff will be required to present new information learned at a monthly in-service presentation.
   g. Assessment by home health, nursing home, and other personnel receiving discharged patients—Scores on feedback forms from agencies receiving patients after discharge will fall within the minimal acceptable range. Items will include promptness of delivery of the patient record; thoroughness of the record, particularly in relation to history, treatment, and status; clarity of goals; and so forth.
2. To function efficiently

   Data regarding the following items will be collected and evaluated:
   a. Length of time from referral to evaluation
   b. Length of time of patient evaluations
   c. Length of time from evaluation to chart documentation
   d. Length of time from patient discharge to recording discharge summary
   e. Individual and collective percentage of time chargeable to patients

   f. Average time for specific procedures
   g. Number of individual patients seen per day by therapists
3. To fiscally operate within the budget
   a. Meet an established budget target.
   b. Meet separate fiscal targets for inpatient versus outpatient operations.
4. To provide excellent clinical education
   a. Student ratings, according to tabulation of exit questionnaires completed by students at the end of their clinical education experience, will be satisfactory or better.
   b. Faculty Coordinators of Clinical Education ratings of clinical education experiences will be satisfactory or better.
   c. Students will meet 80 percent of established student goals.
5. To provide opportunity for staff development
   a. The department will conduct 12 in-service programs during the year.
   b. Average attendance at in-service programs will be 70 percent of available staff.
   c. All full-time staff will be eligible to attend off-campus continuing education programs with financial support from the department.
   d. Sixty percent of eligible staff will attend off-campus continuing education courses.
   e. The departmental policy for promotion from within the department will be followed and required activities documented.
   f. Formal work-performance evaluations will be conducted for each employee twice annually.
   g. Performance deficits, as determined by the work-performance evaluation, will result in a formal plan of remediation for the employee with direct support from the department.

Concluding Thoughts

Although the preceding itemization of subobjectives is far from complete, these samples demonstrate how the use of measurable subobjectives can contribute to validity in assessing success or failure in attaining a primary objective which, standing alone, cannot be measured. Courtesy cannot be measured, but its presence or absence may be reasonably determined by term of address, tone of voice, and choice of vocabulary. The key to writing worthwhile objectives, therefore, is to identify and quantify those factors that allow one to recognize success or failure in attaining the objective.

As with problem solving, the careful differentiation of target objectives is critical. The true task in writing measurable objectives is the proper framing of the process of evaluation. In this case, an assessment of the extent to which departmental objectives are met will be made by the evaluation of the strategies used to achieve those objectives.

ANALYSIS: CASE 9

I DESERVE A MERIT INCREASE

Information Required and Strategies for Gathering Information

Question 1—What Can Be Learned from a Review of Formal Documents?

Strategy: Ms. Martinez will review in detail all work-performance evaluations (WPEs), performance improvement (PI) reports, and personnel records pertaining to Mr. Stone. She will conduct a random check on Mr. Stone's patient records to ascertain the following:

1. Tangible data
   a. Attendance
   b. Punctuality
   c. Billing—timeliness and accuracy
   d. Patient documentation—timeliness
   e. External reports—timeliness
2. Intangible data
   a. Patient documentation—accuracy, thoroughness, clarity
   b. External reports—clarity/thoroughness
   c. Supervisory skills—efficiency, effectiveness, tact

Question 2—What Is Mr. Thomas's Perception of Mr. Stone?

Strategy: Ms. Martinez will have a private, confidential discussion with Mr. Thomas regarding:

1. Mr. Stone's work performance
2. The two most recent WPEs of Mr. Stone
3. Mr. Stone's team leader
4. The relationship between Mr. Stone and his team leader

Question 3—What Is the Perception of Certain Physicians and Other Coworkers of Mr. Stone's Professional Competency?

Strategy: Identify several physicians whose patients are often treated by Mr. Stone ask for their confidential appraisal of Mr. Stone. Also interview coworkers.

Information Gathered

Question 1

On reviewing Mr. Stone's WPEs, Ms. Martinez found that in each of the past 2 years his team leader rated 10 of 11 items as "3" (meets job expectations but does not exceed them) and rated him higher only in the area of patient rapport. Looking back to Mr. Stone's WPE on his first team, Ms. Martinez observed ratings that in almost every case were higher than "3."

1. Tangible data
   a. Attendance—Other than for vacation and approved leave for professional conferences, Mr. Stone was absent only 1 day in 2 years. The average number of absences for other members of his team was 3 days per year.
   b. Punctuality—There were no citations for tardiness. Two other members of the team had several citations each.
   c. Billing—No citations for delay or inaccuracy in billing
   d. Patient documentation—All charts checked indicated timely recording, and there were no citations for delay in any of the reports.
   e. External reports—Random check of such reports failed to identify evidence of delay.
2. Intangible data
   a. Patient documentation—Generally of high standards, consistent and effective use of quantitative measures, measurable goals, clear and thorough.
   b. External reports—Consistent with prior documentation, clearly written and with logical sequence, thorough.
   c. Supervision—Ms. Martinez recalled a number of favorable comments emanating from assistants and aides referring to Mr. Stone's being respectful and giving clear instructions; she could recall no unfavorable comments.

Question 2—Mr. Thomas's Perception

a. Mr. Stone's work performance—Mr. Thomas indicated that he had been favorably impressed with his direct but limited observation of Mr. Stone. He was unaware of any problems.
b. Recent WPEs—Mr. Thomas admitted he was somewhat surprised. He indicated that before approving the latest WPE as presented to him by the team leader he had questioned the rating since his direct observations led him to believe Mr. Stone was exceeding expectation in a number of areas. Mr. Thomas signed the WPE after being told by the team leader that "Mr. Stone was inconsistent—sometimes very good, and other times below expectations." Mr. Thomas recalled suggesting that in the future such remarks be included in the comment section of the form if that were the case.
c. The team leader—Mr. Thomas referred to his work performance evaluations of the team leader and noted that his overall rating was very high. He perceived her to be bright, enthusiastic, efficient, and popular with her team. He had no reason to believe she was anything but fair with her personnel. He had received no complaints about her ability or supervision.
d. Relationship of team leader and Mr. Stone—Mr. Thomas indicated that until this occasion he had no indication of the existence of a problem or

any sort of bias. He stated that Mr. Stone had never complained, nor had anyone else ever indicated friction between them.

Question 3—Other Personnel's Perceptions of Mr. Stone's Professional Competence

Ms. Martinez interviewed five physicians, several nurses, and an occupational therapist who work closely with Mr. Stone and heard nothing but compliments of Mr. Stone. All were impressed with his knowledge, the results he got with patients, his tact and persuasiveness when recommending a program change or in disagreement. Each of them expressed respect for Mr. Stone and the hope that he was not considering leaving the department. None had any complaints.

The analysis of information is quite revealing in that it brings to the foreground a number of significant inconsistencies. With the exception of "patient rapport," which was rated "5" on a 6-point scale, all items on Mr. Stone's two most recent WPEs were rated "3" (meets but does not exceed job expectations). The numerical ratings for the past 2 years were much lower than those recorded previously on another team. Assignment to a new team may contribute to a lower WPE rating the first year, but does not explain the identical rating the second year. Furthermore, the specific tangible and intangible information gathered appear to be in conflict with the WPE ratings.

For example, it is difficult to reconcile a "3" rating for "attendance" when the individual has been absent only 1 day in 2 years, particularly when the average for the team is three absences per person per year! A "3" also seems incompatible with no citations for tardiness or delays in billing, or with consistent, timely documentation and external communication. Ms. Martinez perceived that there was a high standard of patient documentation and that external reports were clear, thorough, and consistent with prior documentation. However high the standards might be in this department, Ms. Martinez's perception of Mr. Stone's performance in these areas is clearly indicative of ratings higher than "3."

Mr. Thomas expressed surprise at the mediocre WPE of Mr. Stone. Although questioning it, he did not pursue the matter further because of his high regard for the team leader as a supervisor and because he had no complaints of bias from Mr. Stone or any other reports of friction between the two. Finally, five physicians and other hospital staff members, whose judgment Ms. Martinez trusted, unanimously offered praise for Stone's professional competency to a degree that loudly suggests exceeding job expectations.

It would not be unreasonable at this point for a manager to conclude that the analysis of the assembled information supports Mr. Stone's contention that his most recent WPE was inaccurate. If Ms. Martinez accepts this conclusion she will redefine the problem and recognize that she now has two problems. The first problem relates to a possible adjustment for Mr. Stone, and the second problem relates to the underlying reason for the team leader's inaccurate assessment of Mr. Stone. Ms. Martinez, who did a commendable job of collecting relevant information, may determine that the information was limited in scope because one of her goals was to avoid a confrontation with the team leader. She may choose to return to Step 3 and gather additional information from one additional source, the team leader.

Concluding Thoughts

This case revolves around the complaint of a staff-level therapist who believes his work performance was rated inaccurately, resulting in the subsequent denial of a merit raise for the second consecutive year. A complaint of this type is not uncommon, particularly in a large department such as the one at Bella Vista Hospital. In fact, it might be more accurate to state that it would be a rarity for at least one individual in a large department not to feel unappreciated and/or misjudged. A complaint of this nature becomes more emotionally charged when it is accompanied by an allegation of discrimination based on gender, race, or sexual preference. Given the existence of such a complaint, the key to sound management lies in the manner in which the allegation is handled, thus providing the lessons to be learned. In the case of alleged discrimination, many facilities have specific procedures for managing these allegations, and such procedures must be carefully followed by the manager.

In reviewing this case, note the immediate response of Ms. Martinez. At the time of the initial discussion with Mr. Stone it would have been easy for her to simply dismiss the allegation by citing her faith in the assistant director and the team leader. It would have been just as easy to deny Mr. Stone the opportunity to fully express his complaint by referring to the chain of command and sending him back to his team leader or to the assistant director who approved the WPE. She could have listened to Mr. Stone's complaint and gone directly to the team leader or to Mr. Thomas and asked for an explanation. And Ms. Martinez could have chosen the time-honored administrative ploy of listening to Mr. Stone and then delegating the problem to the assistant director with a directive to report back to her. Ms. Martinez, however, chose none of those options.

Ms. Martinez allowed Mr. Stone to express his complaint, an allegation of unfair performance appraisal, with no prejudgment of the credibility of the allegation. She did not demonstrate the administrative knee jerk response of supporting management, nor did she accept Mr. Stone's allegation as valid. Ms. Martinez frankly admitted she was not well informed about the details of the WPE, but pledged to look into the matter, discuss it with Mr. Thomas, and get back to him as soon as possible. It is important to note that Ms. Martinez fulfilled her pledge in all respects, demonstrating an important attribute of a respected leader.

Ms. Martinez launched a subtle and nonconfrontational investigation. Directly approaching the team leader runs the risk of causing a number of negative outcomes. These include offending the team leader, shaking the team leader's confidence, offending the assistant director by bypassing him, and possibly causing open hostility between Mr. Stone and his team leader. Ms. Martinez's approach included consultation with Mr. Thomas and postponed or, depending on the findings, prevented confrontation with the team leader.

It should be noted that despite the imposed limitations of a low-profile investigation, Ms. Martinez did a relatively thorough review. She used to advantage existing formal records and other documentation to collect and analyze both tangible and intangible items relating to the WPE. She reviewed objective and quantifiable data relating to attendance, punctuality, and timeliness of various procedures. In the intangible category she made personal assessments relative to documentation and supervision, and she secured the performance assessments of knowledgeable and credible physicians and staff.

Not surprisingly, after gathering and analyzing the information, Ms. Martinez arrived at a fork in the road and was bound to ask, "What next?" Because of the existence of indisputable evidence (attendance, punctuality, and timeliness of billing and reporting) that supported Mr. Stone's allegation, Ms. Martinez had to choose one of two roads, highlighted by these questions:

1. Given the evidence to date, do I now seek additional information and include direct discussion with the team leader?
2. Do I consider the information to be sufficient enough to make a judgement that Mr. Stone has been unfairly treated and therefore proceed to redefine the problem?

An experienced manager is not dismayed or daunted by forks in the road to problem resolution. It is not regarded as a shortcoming or failure when a manager encounters a dilemma as did Ms. Martinez. Had the original problem been perceived and defined differently, the path to resolution might have been more straightforward. The more important lesson to be gained, however, is that no administrator is omniscient and able to unfailingly compose unassailable problem statements. No administrator, therefore, need apologize for occasionally recognizing the wisdom of returning to Step 3 to gather more information or to significantly redefine the problem in Step 5.

ANALYSIS: CASE 10

RIGHT-SIZING

In this case hospital administration, faced with a 10 percent budget deficit in the approaching fiscal year, elected to eliminate that deficit by requiring all departments to reduce their respective budgets by 10 percent. On the surface this seems to be an equitable approach and indeed may have been the best of the options identified by the administration. At the department level, particularly in one that is personnel-oriented, the edict to reduce a budget by 10 percent becomes very personalized; therefore, deciding specifically which persons to discharge demands great deliberation. Unless the manager approaches the issue with a philosophy of "last hired—first fired" or is restricted by policy, many factors and values will influence the resolution of the problem.

The authors call to the attention of the reader the different types of information targeted by Rick Fallon and his associates that reflect greater concern for people than numbers. In the personnel category there was consideration of personal issues such as the "breadwinner" status of individuals; the imminent plans of individuals relating to relocation or return to graduate school, resulting in self-imposed departure; and the specific requirements and qualifications for certain necessary and highly specialized programs.

In the service area there was interest in recent trends and developments as they may affect genuine needs or a diminution of need; quality patient care; the impact of service on the average length of stay in the hospital (an item of critical importance to the administration); and consideration of the relinquishment or shifting of service to another department. In times of growth most budgets include a generous amount for purchase of major equipment (capital expenditures), but in times of recession, capital expenditures may be put on hold. In this case, the postponement of capital expenditures may prove to be a source of funds to salvage one or two personnel positions.

Perhaps the most important lesson to be learned from this case is the importance of identifying all the information that relates to the problem. Careful analysis of this information will enable the manager to develop a more comprehensive list of viable alternatives and enhance the prospects of an effective resolution of the problem. Answering the question about future right-sizing for the service needs of the medical center may be the most visionary place to begin.

ANALYSIS: CASE 11

BIAS AND PREJUDICE

Angela Morelli realized that the kind of information required to resolve her newly stated problem was quite different from that required to resolve her original problem. After much thought Ms. Morelli determined that the following information was needed:

1. On average, how many patients with Alzheimer's disease are treated each day?
2. More specifically, of the patients with Alzheimer's disease, how many of them exhibit symptoms of severely impaired short-term memory and lack of motivation?
3. Is it possible to avoid scheduling Ms. Harris with patients with Alzheimer's disease without being unfair to Ms. Bridges and/or other staff or disrupting normal activity?
4. What is the current state of the supply and demand of PTs in the area? Can Ms. Harris be readily replaced?
5. Is there appropriate counseling available to Ms. Harris to help her overcome her problem?
6. Will Ms. Harris be willing to undergo professional counseling to overcome her problem?
7. Will Ms. Bridges be willing to reschedule an increased number of patients with Alzheimer's disease for a few months? Indefinitely?

As this case developed, Ms. Morelli did acquire the information indicated above and proceeded from there to develop the following list of alternatives:

1. Complete a formal work-performance evaluation citing the bias and placing Ms. Harris on probation with the notice to improve or be terminated.
2. Require Ms. Harris to undergo professional counseling.
3. Plan a "weaning" program in which Ms. Harris would initially be exposed only to those patients with mild symptoms with gradually increasing exposure to those with more severe symptoms of memory and motivation.
4. Avoid scheduling any patients with Alzheimer's disease with Ms. Harris.
5. Request Ms. Harris's resignation immediately.
6. Request Ms. Harris's resignation, allowing time for her to make other arrangements.
7. Serve Ms. Harris with formal notice of termination, with sufficient time for her to make other arrangements.

Concluding Thoughts

The manner in which Ms. Morelli dealt with the situation provides several valuable lessons in problem solving. The first relates to Ms. Morelli's original dilemma concerning the allegations of Ms. Harris's inappropriate treatment of several patients. She stated her problem as, "How do I verify the possibility of an attitudinal bias?" She recognized that she possessed limited information, but rather than waste time and place patients in jeopardy, Ms. Morelli chose to tactfully confront Ms. Harris. This direct approach proved to be very fruitful and enabled her to get to the heart of the matter. Regrettably, many managers avoid the direct approach, finding it awkward or unpleasant. This case demonstrates the potential benefit of a confrontal approach, particularly when executed with tact and sincerity.

This case, like a number of others in this compilation, demonstrates the need at Step 5 to revisit the original statement. The information acquired by Ms. Morelli completely eliminated the need to pursue the original problem statement; however, that same information resulted in the awareness of a new problem. Another key point in problem solving should not be ignored. The necessity of developing a new problem statement results in the necessity to gather new and different information before proceeding.

The final lesson to be derived from this case is that values related to patients and employees influence the formation of alternatives. The consideration of the alternatives and the weighing of the positive and negative factors associated with each alternative will also be influenced by those values.

ANALYSIS: CASE 12

THE ULTIMATUM

The gathering of relevant information preparatory to solving a problem is always important. In this case, gathering information assumes even greater importance because the decision made by Ms. Jones would affect her entire department and could have a tidal-wave effect throughout the organization. Ms. Jones must also be mindful of the potentially negative reactions that may follow her decision. A degree of preparation and organization is required before implementing the investigation or information-gathering process. Because there are so many questions to be formulated and answered, it is necessary to divide the needed information into two categories—fiscal and human.

Fiscal Questions

1. What is the current salary of team leader A?
2. How does team leader A's salary compare with the other team leaders?
3. When did team leader A last receive a salary increment?
4. What was the amount of team leader A's last increment?
5. Will the granting of a 15 percent increment to team leader A result in a chain reaction among the other team leaders?
6. How do the salaries of the team leaders as a group compare with similar positions within the geographic area?
7. If I accede to the 15 percent request for team leader A, how will this affect the increment pool for the other team leaders? Should the extra 5 percent for team leader A be obtained by reducing the increases allocated for the other team leaders?
8. Can the increased increments for all the team leaders be absorbed through projected revenues?
9. How efficacious, fiscally and politically, is it at this time to increase the personnel budget by a wide margin?
10. Is it efficacious to implement increases in fees to accommodate larger increments for all team leaders?
11. What is the potential impact on team A's revenue generation if team leader A should leave?

Human Resource Questions

1. Is there a promising replacement for team leader A among the staff?
2. If the response to 1 is affirmative, how readily can the vacated staff position be filled?
3. If the response to 1 is negative, what are the prospects for successful recruitment of a team leader from an external source?
4. If the 15 percent increment is granted to team leader A without commensurate increases for the other team leaders, what is the probable reaction of the latter?
5. What is the probable reaction of the other team leaders if the 15 percent increment request is denied and team leader A resigns?
6. What is the probable reaction of the members of team A if
   a. The 15 percent increment is granted?
   b. The 15 percent increment request is denied and team leader A resigns?

Some managers may consider the request of team leader A to be an ultimatum (which of course it is, however politely presented) and would choose to reject team leader A's offer out of hand as a matter of principle. The authors suggest that those with such an inclination might be wise to look beyond the implied threat of resignation and consider the circumstances and the spirit of the offer. After all, one can hardly be blamed for being attracted by a 25 percent pay increase.

Answers to the questions posed in Step 3 have not been provided in this case. The emphasis here is on the determination of the information necessary to arrive at a sound decision. Nevertheless, the reader is encouraged to follow the process through the succeeding steps. By doing so the reader will discern that the decision maker in this case is likely to experience mental and emotional anguish along the way.

Step 4, the analysis of the factual and surmised information gathered, might cause some managers to "shoot from the hip" and jump to a conclusion without consideration of the intervening steps. On the other hand, some managers may wish to redefine the problem. "Because I want to retain the services of team leader A and maintain harmony among the other team leaders, what is the best way to increase the budget to accommodate a 15 percent pay increment for team leader A with commensurate increments for the others?" The authors suggest that the first response is inappropriate and the second premature. It is not unreasonable, given certain information, to reach a decision to grant the 15 percent request and provide commensurate increments to the other leaders. By doing so, however, the manager creates a new problem to be analyzed and resolved.

As a manger progresses through Steps 7 (Identifying) and 8 (Weighing), the human factors loom even larger and the degree of difficuly expands. It should be readily recognized that Ms. Jones will have extreme difficulty in gathering hard-core, tangible responses to her questions. Therefore, some of the information is certain to be intangible conjecture making it much more difficult to assess than the tangible fiscal issues.

ANALYSIS: CASE 13

KEEPING THE LID ON IT

Ms. Sawyer identified numerous sources of information and support to assist her and her staff with the transition process. She divided her list into four sections.

Personal Contacts

1. Call the headquarters of the American Physical Therapy Association to ask for printed materials, information about APTA activities related to hospital restructuring and patient-focused care, and names of facilities that have successfully completed the restructuring process.
2. Call other directors of rehabilitation across the state to identify individuals at institutions within the state that are currently undergoing this type of restructuring or that have successfully completed the process.

3. Call directors of similar services at the other hospitals in the corporation to obtain information.
4. Call fellow managers at the hospital.

Written Materials

1. Carefully review all written materials provided by the corporation.
2. Research literature on patient-focused care and hospital restructuring at the State Medical Center Library.
3. Study the materials provided by the APTA.
4. Read articles in recent professional journals and newsletters.
5. Review graduate school materials on managing change.
6. Obtain recent popular books on leadership and organizational restructuring from the local bookstore.

Resources for Staff Support

1. Call the hospital's Employee Assistance Program to ask for ideas about ways to support staff through the transition process.
2. Call Human Resources Department to inquire about anticipated job reclassifications, changes in salary scales, implications for full-time or part-time employees, and any other anticipated policy changes.

Information about Respiratory Therapy and Therapeutic Recreation Services

1. Contact current department head of Respiratory and Therapeutic Recreation Services.
2. Study professional literature.

Ms. Sawyer recognized the need to organize the information she collected so that it would be easy to retrieve and share with her staff and management colleagues. She started a binder for the articles she collected and prepared a table of contents to help her keep track of them. She also started a journal in which she entered notes about each of her personal communications and listed ideas, questions, and actions for further consideration. Finally, she developed a timeline for each step of the change process, indicating the opportunities she anticipated for staff input and education along the way.

By the time of the staff meeting Monday morning, Ms. Sawyer was prepared to address her staff with confidence that the change was manageable and provided legitimate opportunities for professional advancement. She was able to listen to their fears without being overwhelmed by them. She explained the timeline and the resource notebook, and she encouraged the staff to collect and add their own information. She scheduled bimonthly meetings to focus on the transition process and asked the department secretary to record and distribute detailed minutes. She then asked two of the staff therapists to review these minutes regularly to be sure that the staff's ideas and concerns were being addressed.

Concluding Thoughts

In addition to general human inertia, fear is usually the major cause of resistance to change. The most useful antidotes for fear are information, assurance that the change can be managed successfully, and involvement of staff in the change process. Managers, who in their role as leaders are often called upon to be agents of change, must be sensitive to the needs and concerns of those affected by the change. Development of specific timelines for the transition process, keeping staff informed throughout the process, and involving staff in decision making at every opportunity are strategies that managers find effective in helping staff adapt. The most successful and easily managed changes are those that originate as a result of problems and solutions identified by the staff, rather than those imposed by a top-down administration. Major organizational restructuring, however, rarely occurs in this manner.

ANALYSIS: CASE 14

VIVE LA DIFFÉRENCE!

In any problem-solving situation it is always beneficial to look beyond the problem to determine its cause. In this particular case a major contributing factor is the job description and the determination of qualifications. Mr. Walsh listed five items. The first three were quantifiable and measurable. The last two were neither quantifiable nor measurable. As the qualifications were stated, an applicant must meet all five criteria to be eligible for the position. Many managers, however, would justifiably place greater priority on the two less tangible items than on the measurable criteria of supervisory experience. Measurable criteria are needed to quickly and unequivocally determine eligibility for a position. Other criteria are needed to rate the eligible applicants. The authors prefer the terminology "required" and "preferred" over the term "qualifications" (Fig. 5).

No candidate who fails to meet the "required" criteria should be considered for the position. Generally speaking, the candidate among those eligible who best meets the "preferred" criteria should be considered the strongest candidate for the position. If at any time the manager wants to appoint or promote an ineligible candidate over the eligible candidates, the manager may be guilty of creating more rigorous criteria

JOB SPECIFICATIONS

I. Required: Include all quantifiable and measurable items considered absolutely essential for job performance and eligibility for the job. Examples include licensure, number of years experience, prior administrative experiences, and specialty certification.

II. Preferred: Include those items beyond basic eligibility that will enhance job performance and favorably influence the applicant's status. These may include quantifiable and measurable items such as a greater number of years experience than is required, or eligibility for certification versus actual certification in a specialty. In addition, and not to be minimized in importance, are the unquantifiable and nonmeasurable factors, including character and work traits such as organizational skills, communication skills, interpersonal attitudes/skills, patience, interest in teaching students, flexibility, leadership skills, and ability to speak a specific language.

FIGURE 5.

than necessary. In this case, for example, was it necessary to require 1 year of supervisory experience?

Concluding Thoughts

The distinction of "required" and "preferred" criteria clarifies the vital issue of job eligibility and significantly reduces the threat of litigation for alleged improper hiring practices. The manager must weigh carefully all items in relation to performance expectations for a job before making a determination of "required" or "preferred." Similarly, the manager must be sure that criteria do not discriminate among applicants based on noncritical job functions. This is particularly important in following the requirements of the Americans with Disabilities Act (ADA), which protects individuals whose disability need not interfere with their ability to perform necessary job functions.

Steps 6–7

Developing Alternative Strategies and Identifying the Positive and Negative Factors of Each

ANALYSIS: CASE 15

MANAGING INVENTORY

Sam and Rob developed the following list of possible actions:

1. Search all employees as they leave.
2. Search patients' bags as they leave.
3. Assign a second person to count towels when sending and receiving laundry.
4. Conduct towel inventory weekly instead of monthly.
5. Raise the matter at staff meeting.

Sam and Rob at first silently mused over the list and then shared their views about each possibility. They were in complete accord all the way through the list. They concluded that a search of each employee would result in resentment, anger, and a serious drop in morale. A search of selective individuals was discriminatory and out of the question. They considered a search of patients' bags a terribly negative public relations move that would have serious impact on their business. They estimated that the extra cost of assigning a second person to count towels would counterbalance or outweigh any reduction in loss that might ensue. Neither Sam nor Rob could identify any particular benefit to doing inventory weekly rather than monthly. They thought there might be some value in alerting the staff about the problem and asking them to be more observant.

Sam and Rob concluded their meeting by agreeing they would mention the recent increase in towel disappearance at the next staff meeting. Otherwise they did nothing but monitor the situation, with plans to review it at a later date.

Concluding Thoughts

In the introduction to this book there was reference to the fact that experienced managers may quickly move through the necessary steps in problem solving, just as they may do in resolving a clinical problem. That was the case with Sam and Rob. They expressed a concern, put that concern into a problem context, identified and analyzed the relevant information, listed alternatives that might lead to resolution, analyzed the alternatives, and weighed the consequences of each. Simply because they did not enumerate and label each step of the process does not detract from the fact that they followed a rational and thorough sequence of activities leading to the final step of making a choice.

In the final analysis Sam and Rob selected an alternative not initially identified—namely, do nothing! There are times when the manager may rightfully determine that (1) none of the alternatives is viable, (2) the cost of even the most viable alternative outweighs the benefit to be derived, (3) the problem is not of sufficient magnitude to justify implementation of the alternatives, or (4) the problem is likely to quickly resolve itself or be resolved by its rightful owner. For example, if one's automobile fuel tank leaks one drop per week, the leakage is not a safety risk nor worth the cost of repair. On the other hand, if the tank is losing a gallon per week, the tank should be repaired for safety and financial reasons. In the case of the missing towels, Sam and Rob did not find the problem to be of sufficient magnitude to implement any of the alternatives other than advising the staff of the situation.

Most people look for and respect decisiveness on the part of managers. There are times, however, when it is appropriate to do nothing about a situation. Inaction as a conscious choice must be recognized as a decision and distinguished from failure to respond.

ANALYSIS: CASE 16

ALLOCATION OF MERIT INCREMENTS

Step 1—Recognizing

Is there a problem in need of a decision? There is a problematic situation in that Mr. Crown has a specific amount of money that may be used for merit increments for three supervisors who received different work-performance evaluations (WPEs). The decision must be made because of the deadline for submitting a proposed budget, including the merit awards.

Step 2—Defining

Mr. Crown has the opportunity to reward his supervisors with salary increases for meritorious service within a cap of $6400. Which, if any, of the supervisors should receive an increment, and how much?

Step 3—Investigating

1. **WPEs.** Supervisor A achieved a much higher rating than her colleagues, and supervisor C was rated far below A and B in most items.
2. **Nonrated information.** Supervisor A seems to have the most innate talent for the position, and her team outperformed the others by a wide margin. Supervisor C has the least experience in the position and less innate talent, but he gets the most from his potential and tries very hard.
3. **Salaries.** In fact, there is not a wide spread between the highest and lowest of the three salaries, with "A" receiving only 12.5 percent more than "C" despite greater longevity in the position.
4. **Increment pool.** Mr. Crown has a pool of $6400 that he can allocate to any or all of the three supervisors. The individual caps for supervisors A, B, and C are $4500, $4300, and $4000, respectively.

Step 4—Analyzing

The information in this case is relatively straightforward. Current salaries are consistent with seniority and with the work-performance ratings of the three supervisors. According to the WPEs, there is no question as to the relative performance of the three, although there is a suggestion that supervisor A, despite the highest rating and top team performance, is capable of even more. Supervisor B, although not rated as high as supervisor A, received ratings of 4 and 5 in all items in the WPE, strongly suggesting performance of higher caliber.

Step 5—Confirming

The problem or opportunity as defined in Step 2 is confirmed.

Step 6—Developing

Many possible alternatives for distributing merit awards exist. The only limitations are the total cap of $6400 and the individual cap of 10 percent per supervisor. For the purpose of this exercise, however, only four models (Figs. 6–9) are presented, representing two middle-of-the-road approaches and two extremes.

Step 7—Identifying

Table 4 outlines the positive and negative factors associated with each alternative.

Concluding Thoughts

The allocation of merit increments ranks among the thorniest of administrative decisions and most troublesome of administrative responsibilities. There is the ever-present potential for major disappointment and resentment among employees. Judi-

ALTERNATIVE 1

Supervisor "A"	10.0%–$4500
Supervisor "B"	4.4%–$1900
Supervisor "C"	0.0%–$ 0

Rationale:

1. Supervisor A received the highest rating in the work performance evaluations.
2. The productivity of supervisor A's team exceeds that of supervisors B and C.
3. Supervisor C failed to demonstrate excellence in at least 2 of the 10 rated items and, subject to interpretation, possibly 4 of the 10; therefore, C does not deserve a merit increment.
4. All of supervisor B's ratings were at the two highest levels, therefore B deserves some tangible recognition.

FIGURE 6.

ALTERNATIVE 2

Supervisor "A"	0.8%–$ 325
Supervisor "B"	5.0%–$2150
Supervisor "C"	10.0%–$4000

Rationale:

1. Supervisor C tries harder than supervisors A and B.
2. Supervisor C functions at his or her maximum potential whereas supervisors A and B do not.
3. Supervisor C has less experience than the others and should not be expected to perform at the same level.
4. This plan tends to balance the three salaries in recognition of equal work/responsibility and prevents a further widening of the salary spread among the three supervisors.
5. Supervisor A exerts the least effort of the three and realizes less of his or her full potential.
6. Supervisors B and C demonstrate better interpersonal attitudes than supervisor A.

FIGURE 7.

cious determination of merit increments demands of the manager a combination of objectivity, wisdom, fairness, and courage, particularly when the available alternatives are as diverse as in this case.

A review of the four alternative plans confirms the significant differences among them, particularly from the one extreme to the other. Each alternative has the potential to offend one or more of the supervisors. Alternative 1, for example, has the potential to offend supervisor C, who will not receive a merit increment. Conversely, it is supervisor A who will be offended by Alternative 2 in view of the al-

ALTERNATIVE 3

Supervisor "A"	05.0%–$2250
Supervisor "B"	05.0%–$2150
Supervisor "C"	05.0%–$2000

Rationale:

1. Despite individual differences in the WPEs, all three supervisors deserve an increment.
2. Supervisor A's increase is suitable reward in that his or her 5% increment results in a greater dollar reward.
3. This plan maintains the relative balance of salaries among the three. Longevity and performance are rewarded with larger dollar increments but not to the significant detriment of supervisor C.
4. This is a relatively "safe" plan. None of the supervisors is likely to become upset.

FIGURE 8.

ALTERNATIVE 4

Supervisor "A"	04.74%–$2133
Supervisor "B"	04.96%–$2133
Supervisor "C"	05.33%–$2133

Rationale:

1. Items 1, 3, and 4 from **Alternative 3** apply to this plan as well.
2. Because each of the supervisors receives an arbitrary 3% increment in addition to the merit increment, supervisors A and B receive greater monetary rewards than C.

FIGURE 9.

most nonexistent merit increment despite a high WPE rating. Although Alternatives 3 and 4 might be considered "safer" in terms of offending any of the supervisors, supervisors A and B will not be overjoyed by either of these alternatives.

The authors suggest that in the final analysis it is the value system of the manager that will greatly influence the ultimate determination of merit increments. The authors also suggest that the manager is entitled to use values as a guide in making decisions providing the manager's values are not in conflict with organizational values. It is critical, however, that the manager inform subordinates of those values from the outset of the evaluation period. In this case, the manager should make clear to all staff his values relative to performance versus effort. If particular items hold greater value in the appraisal of work performance, those items should be weighted accordingly in the WPE form.

TABLE 4
Positive and Negative Factors for Each Alternative

Positive Factors	Negative Factors
Alternative 1	
Supervisors A and B are likely to be satisfied and motivated to maintain high quality performance.	Supervisor C very probably will be disappointed and discouraged.
The best-performing supervisor is less likely to look for "greener pastures."	Supervisor C may experience a drop in performance because of discouragement and lack of confidence.
Provides a clear message to all members of the department that performance will be rewarded.	Supervisor C may explore other employment opportunities.
Alternative 2	
Supervisors B and C are likely to be satisfied, particularly C.	Supervisor A is most likely to be very unhappy and resentful.
Provides a clear message to all members of the department that effort and positive interpersonal behavior will be rewarded.	There is a distinct possibility that supervisor A may look elsewhere for employment and/or lower her level of performance.
	Supervisors B and C may become complacent.
Alternative 3	
Hopefully, none of the supervisors will be greatly unhappy.	Supervisor A is likely to be disappointed.
Provides a message to all staff that both performance and effort will be rewarded.	Supervisor B may be uncertain as to the basis of his increment—performance or equality?
Supervisor C should feel very gratified and continue to strive to improve his skills.	
The existing salary spread is maintained.	
Alternative 4	
Positive and negative factors for Alternative 3 also apply to 4.	

ANALYSIS: CASE 17

OH! THE FRUSTRATION OF IT ALL

There are times when a single possibility may be expected to have sufficient impact to resolve the problem; however, that is not always the case. In the absence of a single problem-solving alternative, it may be necessary to identify a number of less potent alternatives whose combined effect may result in resolution. In this case the list of potential strategies is lengthy and diverse. One way to organize them is to separate group or collective strategies from individual strategies. Listed below are a number of the possible strategies to be considered for implementation.

Individual Strategies

Ms. Bryant

1. Convince a patient to file a formal complaint.
2. Encourage occupational therapy (OT) staff to document all nursing deficiencies in patients' charts.
3. Report nursing deficiencies to third-party payers.
4. Notify local news media of deficiencies.
5. Extend an olive branch to Ms. Hurley, indicate that she will exert pressure for additional nursing staff if Ms. Hurley will guarantee better service if staff is increased.
6. Send a memo to Mr. Bacon, with copies to the president and vice president of patient care, deploring the quality of nursing care for patients and emphasizing the potential threat of litigation resulting from below-standard care.

OT Staff

1. Thorough documentation in patient's charts of all instances of Nursing's lack of compliance with treatment plan.
2. Report all cases of noncompliance to patient representative.

Medical Director

1. Cite all cases of nursing noncompliance in reports of Performance Improvement Committee.
2. Approach the administration with strong request for additional nursing staff.

Physical Therapy (PT) Department

1. Support OT with medical staff and administration.
2. Document noncompliance

Patient Representative

1. Exercise authority of the position to demand compliance.
2. Provide patients with a more thorough orientation as to their rights.
3. Notify the administration of noncompliance and the potential threat of litigation from families of patients.

Collective Strategies

1. Implement a concerted effort on the part of all involved disciplines to document all instances of noncompliance in the charts of the patients affected.
2. Organize a coordinated effort to support Ms. Hurley in her efforts to improve the staff/patient ratio in the nursing service.
3. Threaten the administration with a plan to "go public" with the deficiencies in nursing care.

The list of strategies as presented above, and as perhaps developed by individual readers, contains a number of drastic steps. As these alternatives are analyzed and weighed, some will be rejected. It is the view of the authors that, despite the intensity of concern for patient care and the high level of frustration experienced by Ms. Byrant, some measures are more likely to have negative rather than positive effects and should not be selected at this time. These include:

1. Persuading a patient to file a formal complaint
2. Either singularly or collectively "going public"
3. Notification of third-party payers of noncompliance

Convincing a patient to file a formal complaint would not only destroy the patient's confidence in RRC and the treatment being provided, but it would open the door for litigation against the center and its staff, neither of which is a desirable outcome. Broadcasting RRC's problems to either the local news media or third-party payors has the potential of effecting positive changes in the long run; however, the probable short-term effects could be devastating to RRC. If such action was undertaken by Ms. Bryant individually, there is a strong possibility of a boomerang effect in which resentment could be directed at her by the administration and others, thus rendering her even less effective.

The strategies likely to have the greatest impact are those in which there is coordination and unity of action across departments and services. Consolidated efforts by medicine, OT, PT, and the patient representative to improve the staff/patient ratio in nursing would appear to be a commendable and successful strategy.

Concluding Thoughts

A significant lesson to be learned from this case is the evolution of different problem statements as Ms. Bryant worked through the problem-solving process. Of particular importance is the revision of the perception of Ms. Hurley. In the beginning she was, in effect, perceived as the root of the problem. With the collection and analysis of information, however, there develops an awareness and appreciation of Ms. Hurley's plight and a new perception of her as a fellow victim. It is this type of transformation that lends credence to a systematic and thorough problem-solving approach.

ANALYSIS: CASE 18

PLEASE SAY "I DON'T KNOW"

This case illustrates the thin line that exists between the benefits to be derived from being confident and independent and the inherent danger associated with being overconfident and blind to one's limitations. This case also demonstrates the acuity of Mr. Breen who recognized and accepted his responsibility as a supervisor and was willing to confront a sensitive situation. Also demonstrated in this case is the open line of communication between supervisor and department head and their mutual concern for patients and the organization. It is this mutual concern that resulted in the formal recognition of a problem.

Some who review this case may fault Mr. Breen and Ms. Finnegan for waiting too long before taking decisive action. It is not difficult to condemn such a delay. There are, however, two major arguments against hasty action. First, the cost, in time and money, associated with the recruitment and orientation of a professional employee is high; therefore, reasonable effort to salvage the situation is indicated. Second, there was ample evidence in this case that Mr. Talbott did have the potential to become an excellent physical therapist. It was, therefore, a sound investment of time to give him the opportunity to reach that potential.

The reader's assignment was to develop a list of available alternatives to resolve the problem and to identify and weigh the positive and negative factors associated with each alternative. All or most of the following alternatives should have been identified:

Alternative	*Positive Factors*	*Negative Factors*
Ignore the problem and do nothing. Hope Mr. Talbott matures over time.	The problem of recruitment is eliminated.	The issues of quality care remain.
Have Mr. Talbott seek professional counseling.	A positive change may result.	This may simply delay the inevitable; potential danger still exists.
Place Mr. Talbott on suspension without pay until he seeks professional counseling and acknowledges his errors of omission and commission.	Danger is eliminated.	This is costly to Talbott; it disturbs schedules.
Formally extend Mr. Talbott's period of probation an additional 3 months.	Mr. Talbott is given opportunity to change; UHHA retains option for instant termination.	Concerns for quality of care remain.
Place in writing an ultimatum of termination of employment if there is one more episode involving his failure to recognize his limitations and request assistance.	Clarifies status for Talbott while giving him one more chance simplifies termination process for UHHA if he does not chance.	Threat could have negative effect on Mr. Talbott's performance.
Terminate Mr. Talbott's employment immediately.	Eliminates the problem and potential danger to patients.	New problems of recruitment and scheduling.

The weight given to the positive and negative factors associated with each alternative will vary with the individual manager. As stated previously, the manager's unique mix of values, experiences, level of confidence, and other tangible factors (such as supply and demand) all influence the weighing process and guide the manager toward a final decision.

ANALYSIS: CASE 19

ALLOCATION OF LIMITED FISCAL RESOURCES

Ms. Adams, at some point in Steps 6 through 8, will probably experience dissatisfaction with the available alternatives. When the dissatisfaction is strong enough, she will wonder, "Is there another approach?" In fact, there is another possibility. The videostroboscopy unit of choice (cost—$50,000) could be leased for $1150 per month for 1 year with option for purchase at $45,000 at the end of the 12-month period.

A conservative projected utilization rate of the videostroboscopy unit suggests that after the first month, in which the emphasis would be on training of personnel and on marketing, the minimal revenue generated by the unit would be $3000 per month. That amount is more than adequate to pay the rental cost without utilizing any of the $100,000 allocation.

If approval is granted by Mr. Bainbridge, the videostroboscopy unit is no longer a factor in the deliberations. Ms. Adams might then return to Step 6. In effect, she is dealing with a revised request of $130,000 and a shortfall of $30,000.

The reader is encouraged to develop a revised set of alternatives.

Concluding Thoughts

For some problems the difficulty lies not in the identification or development of alternatives, but rather in limiting the alternatives to a reasonable number of a representative variety. Sometimes the manager may not be enamored with any of the alternatives first identified and analyzed. It may prove beneficial for the manager to return to Step 6 and attempt to develop more creative alternatives.

The most controversial factor in this case is most likely the amount of the salary increment. Because staff members were described as "outdated and ultraconservative" and not engaged in continuing education activities, some managers would argue against an appreciable increment. In fact, some managers would oppose any increment at all on the grounds that the staff should first demonstrate changes in attitude and practice before receiving a wage increment. Proponents of elevation of the wage scale by a minimum of 10 percent are likely to argue that staff performance is linked to prior lackluster management and inadequate pay. Furthermore, these advocates might point out that this is a golden opportunity. This may be the only opportunity to adjust salaries to a level that will greatly enhance recruitment of personnel in the future.

Ms. Adams was the sole problem solver in this case. Advocates of a participatory style of management might suggest staff involvement throughout the process of problem solving. The advantage of a participatory process is the diffusion of staff dissatisfaction and shared ownership in the solution. The danger of involving staff in this case is their predictable bias related to salary increases, but staff involvement should not be automatically eliminated. If a participatory approach is implemented, however, it must be done with great caution. Specific limitations may be imposed by Ms. Adams to balance the natural bias harbored by the staff. If staff participation is to be employed, Ms. Adams might first ask for a specific commitment from staff to develop contemporary knowledge and skills regardless of the alternative selected.

Steps 8–10

Weighing and Choosing Alternatives and Evaluating the Outcome

ANALYSIS: CASE 20

PROMOTE FROM WITHIN OR HIRE FROM OUTSIDE

Step 1—Recognizing

Is there a need to make a decision? Yes, because the assistant director has resigned and Ms. Brown has determined the need to maintain the position.

Step 2—Defining

Which of the two most highly rated candidates should be selected to fill the position of assistant director?

Step 3—Investigating

Ms. Brown has gathered and organized relevant information.

Step 4—Analyzing

This too was done by Ms. Brown.

Step 5—Confirming

The issue is not simply a matter of choosing between the two finalists for the position. A more insightful approach might be to analyze the greatest positive impact and/or least negative impact on the department achieved by the appointment of either of the two final candidates.

Step 6—Developing

Ms. Brown developed alternatives by reducing the field to two candidates, one internal and the other external.

Step 7—Identifying

Ms. Brown identified the positive and negative factors associated with each choice in a tentative way.

Step 8—Weighing

Ms. Brown arrived at a critical point in the process because she could only speculate about the potential impact of her choices. She has insufficient information to complete this step. If she is to make a decision in the best interest of her department, Ms. Brown must go back to Steps 3 and 4 to gather and analyze information pertaining to the following:

1. The probable reaction of the internal candidate to the appointment of the external candidate
2. The probable reaction of the staff to the appointment of either candidate
3. The impact on the sports program if the senior physical therapist is promoted or if she resigns if not promoted

Concluding Thoughts

In analyzing this case there are two primary lessons to be learned. The first lesson relates to the gathering of information. It is important to note that although Ms. Brown had done a creditable job of gathering and analyzing information, her initial effort was insufficient to enable her to make the best choice. She found she had to go from Step 8 back to Steps 3 and 4 to gather additional information. To fail to do so would have resulted in the selection of an assistant director based largely on credentials and intuition as to the staff's reaction. It is not uncommon, nor necessarily an indication of poor preparation, for an able manager to recognize the need for additional information. In this case it is essential to make an accurate assessment of staff reaction to the appointment of the external candidate over the popular, but less experienced, colleague. Furthermore, Ms. Brown must develop an accurate appraisal concerning the impact on the sports physical therapy program, no matter which of the two candidates is selected.

The second lesson to be gained is that however objective a manager may strive to be, many personnel decisions involve more than such tangible factors as years or type of experience. In addition to being influenced by staff reaction to a given choice, Ms. Brown will be influenced by her own and the hospital's values and priorities as they relate to upward mobility for staff, equal opportunity, and choosing the best-qualified candidate for a position.

The "problem or opportunity" as originally perceived was redefined in Step 5, appropriately changing the emphasis from the simple choice of the better of two candidates to the more complex consideration of what is best for the department. There are times when the statements may result in the same choice, but not always. The effective manager must be prepared to cope with the potential conflict between different responses to interrelated problems.

ANALYSIS: CASE 21

THE UNWANTED ASSIGNMENT

The focus of this case is not on the problem itself, but rather on the catch-all clause, which clearly resolved Ms. Barwell's problem and created Mr. Jordan's. A thoughtful examination of the phrase, "and any other activity assigned by the immediate supervisor or the director" clarifies the all-encompassing nature of the statement and the total authority of the immediate supervisor or the director. The employee must comply with any assigned activity or face the consequences. To say the least, it is a powerful statement, and for better or worse many organizations routinely include such a statement in their job descriptions.

There are several major arguments for the inclusion of a catch-all clause in the job description. The first is based on the premise that it is too unwieldy to include each individual job duty and responsibility within the job-description document. A second argument recognizes that individuals may rotate assignments within the department (such as rotating from one service to another) and although the basic nature of the position may remain the same, there are individual differences. A third argument suggests that it is impossible to anticipate all changes that might occur within a department, whether internally or externally motivated, which may affect the job. And fourth, for the sake of effective and efficient management, the supervisor's ability to assign duties must be maintained.

Some managers purposely do not include a catch-all clause in their job descriptions for professional personnel, relying instead on the professional maturity and integrity of personnel to respond positively to sound leadership. The two main arguments these administrators invoke against the catch-all clause are

1. The employee is placed in a defenseless position, completely at the mercy of the supervisor and with no recourse.
2. The clause in question opens the door for abuse by the supervisor, particularly in any situation in which bias or personal antagonism exists.

To place this issue in its proper perspective, it may be helpful to examine the job description in terms of purpose and format. There are three major purposes of the job description: (1) to define the job and its qualifications for the purpose of recruitment and selection of personnel, (2) to clarify expected work activity and administrative authority, and (3) to serve as a basis for work-performance evaluation.

Job-description formats vary as a result of an organization's style, philosophy, or unique mission and goals. Some job descriptions are overly lengthy and detailed, while others are too brief to be of value. Terminology varies from one organization to another. The criteria by which a candidate will be judged may be labeled as "requirements," "qualifications," "minimal prerequisites," or any of several other designations. The terminology used is not as important as the extent to which the format fulfills the three purposes for which the job description will be used. The authors recommend the format modified from Feitelberg* (Fig. 10).

RECOMMENDED JOB DESCRIPTION FORMAT

I. **Job Title:** i.e., Staff PT; Team Leader; Assistant Director

II. **Immediate Supervisor:** The TITLE of the individual (i.e., Team Leader A; Assistant Director; Director)

III. **Job Summary:** A brief sentence or phrase providing an overview of the job
Example 1 for staff PT—To provide evaluation and treatment for assigned patients
Example 2 for Orthopedic Team Leader—To coordinate and supervise the activities of PTs and other personnel assigned to the orthopedic team

IV. **Job Activities:** Major activities associated with the position
A. *Duties*—Those activities required to be conducted in a specific way as per designated procedure, as
1. Complete and turn in all charge slips to "X" daily
2. Record evaluation and treatment services for each patient daily

B. *Responsibilities*—Those activities for which the individual is accountable but with flexibility and self-determination of method of performance within stated policies, as
1. Evaluate and treat assigned patients
2. Provide clinical education instruction and supervision for three PT students per year
3. Present in-service education programs to team on regular rotating basis

V. **Job Specifications:** To determine (1) eligibility and (2) ranking among applicants for the position
A. *Required*—The tangible and/or measurable minimal standard; that from which there is no deviation or exception; the bottom line, as
1. Licensure as a PT in "X" state
2. 3 years experience as a PT
3. 1 year supervisory experience

B. *Preferred*—That which the employer desires for the position, but may relent or forgive; also intangible and nonmeasurable items as
1. 5 years experience
2. 2 years supervisory experience
3. Effective communication skills
4. Enjoys working with (children, older people, and so forth)

FIGURE 10.

*SB Feitelberg, Basic Considerations of a Job Description. *Journal of the American Physical Therapy Association,* Vol 46, No 4, 1966, pp 383–386.

Return now to the episode in which Ms. Barwell cited the catch-all phrase in the job description. Regardless of the outcome, the evaluation of the decision should include consideration of the Job Activity section of the job description. Two basic issues relate to the specificity and comprehensiveness of the duties and responsibilities outlined and the inclusion of a catch-all clause. There has been no previous employee back injury prevention program in existence. Therefore, that specific responsibility could not have been included in the job description for Mr. Jordan's position or in any other job description. Other potential programs or responsibilities that might arise at some future date are also not included. It is the uncertainty of the future as well as the desire for control that justifies for many the need to include a catch-all clause in job descriptions. The authors respectfully disagree with that premise.

Concluding Thoughts

We consider a catch-all phrase such as the one used in this case excessive and rife with the potential for abuse by a supervisor. Under the terms of that clause, the supervisor or director could demand anything of the individual, including the most menial or unpleasant of tasks. The potential for abuse is greatest in those situations in which bias exists or in which there is a less than positive relationship between supervisor and supervisee. Professional personnel are far more likely to respond favorably to sound leadership and effective communication than to an intimidating clause in a job description.

We recognize that there are managers who are more comfortable with greater authority over employees and therefore prefer to have a control such as a catch-all clause included in the job description. To reduce the potential for abuse, our advice to managers who prefer this approach is to temporize the clause as follows:

> and all other reasonable, professionally related activities consistent with the objectives of the department and with the activities of peers

This modified version precludes the unreasonable demand of menial or debasing activities, and also assures the employee that an excessively heavy workload will not be imposed. It does not, however, assure Mr. Jordan that he can escape responsibility for developing the new program.

ANALYSIS: CASE 22

IS THIS COURSE NECESSARY?

The key to weighing alternatives is the information that is not known, which in this case would include speculation as follows:

1. What is the likelihood of retention of Ms. Denny and Ms. Eaves if
   a. Requests are approved?
   b. Requests are not approved?
   c. For how long?
2. What are the prospects for successful recruitment of replacements if Ms. Denny and/or Ms. Eaves resign?

3. What is the likely effect on the quality and quantity of work produced by Ms. Denny and Ms. Eaves if the requests are approved? Denied?
4. What effect, if any, will the decisions have on the rest of the staff?
5. What are the likely long-term effects on the department if the requests are approved? Denied?
6. What are the possible reactions if one request is approved and the other is denied?

It is critical for the manager in this case to develop perceptions that are as accurate and reliable as possible. If approval of the continuing education requests is denied, will Ms. Denny and Ms. Eaves leave? How easily can they be replaced? Or will they stay, with a diminution in the quantity and quality of work performed? Conversely, if approval is granted, will Ms. Denny and Ms. Eaves be available for another 2 years? Will they, despite different career aspirations, maintain their excellent work performance? Will other staff be resentful of an action that they might perceive as selfish? The answers to these questions will greatly influence the manager as she chooses to either grant or deny these requests.

Concluding Thoughts

In reviewing the case there are two factors that can have a significant influence on the outcome. The first factor is how seriously the manager values the concept of personal development of the individual employee. Although the value of individual employee development is often professed it is ignored in action unless there is an immediate and tangible benefit to the organization. Managers who practice what they profess are likely to cite the intangible benefits that may accrue, such as increased loyalty and the enhancement of the department's reputation as "a good place to work." In these days of intense competition for therapists in a high-demand and low-supply market, a smaller facility not located in an urban area often needs those intangibles to attract and retain staff. The intangible facts of life should not be ignored.

The second major factor that can influence the outcome of this case is that a manager's decisions and actions must be in the long-term best interest of the organization. The manager must weigh the needs of the organization against the needs and desires of individuals. Although the needs and desires of the individual should not be ignored, neither should the needs and interests of the organization. In this particular case, it is reasonable to argue that approval of Ms. Denny's or Ms. Eaves' request will have no tangible detrimental effect on the department and may have a positive long-term benefit. Nevertheless, this argument must be tempered by the consideration of potential future ramifications when making a precedent-setting decision.

ANALYSIS: CASE 23

ONLY A MATTER OF TIME

The use of an external consultant by Ms. Cobb is a strategy to be commended. Not only did she want to add credibility to her allegations about Ms. Chung, but she wanted to be fair. Her explanation to Ms. Chung and offering her a veto in choosing a consultant also are actions to be commended.

The consultant in this case confirmed Ms. Cobb's assessment of the situation and added some insightful information as well. This, of course, was pleasing to Ms. Cobb; however, the rather stark "either/or" recommendation, although reasonable on the surface, seemed less than pleasing to her after her discussion with Ms. Chung. The recommendation provided two alternatives: Ms. Chung's commitment of time for administrative activity would be increased, or she would be replaced. The "replaced," whether interpreted as "terminated" or "demoted," did not sit well with either of the principals.

Earlier in her consideration of the problem, Ms. Cobb did identify another viable alternative. She reasoned that with the growth of the department there was a need for an expert clinician and teacher to work with inexperienced OTs and OT students. She reviewed the department's fiscal status and determined that it could support a new position with joint responsibility for clinical service and clinical teaching. Ms. Cobb immediately approached Mr. Adams with the proposal to replace Ms. Chung as director and appoint her to the new position, with no reduction in salary, if she was willing to accept reassignment. When Mr. Adams approved the plan, Ms. Cobb presented it to Ms. Chung, who thought it was a great idea and accepted the offer enthusiastically.

Concluding Thoughts

The situation described in this case is not unusual. Many individuals enter the health professions because they are people-oriented and harbor a desire to help people in need. Upon graduation from an educational program most young therapists do in fact spend most of their time in direct patient care. With the passage of time a significant percentage of individuals will be promoted to management positions. Others, as in the case of Ms. Chung, begin as director in a small department and lead it through the evolutionary process of growth until the primary role of director changes dramatically. Some make the transition smoothly and effectively with no regrets. Others, like Ms. Chung, continue to view themselves as clinicians first and managers second.

A second point of importance in this case relates to the respective values of both Ms. Chung and Ms. Cobb. Ms. Chung clearly places the highest values on patient service, teaching, and loyalty to the organization. Ms. Cobb seems to place the highest values on sound management, punctuality, and concern for the individual. This is not a case in which values conflict, but rather one in which the priorities do not match. Resolution of a problem in which values are somewhat mismatched is far more probable than when values are totally incompatible.

ANALYSIS: CASE 24

THE WEEKEND RETREAT

Concluding Thoughts

This case focused on the sudden revolt of the physical therapy staff against their director, Tom Gray. This revolt, as often is the case, was not the result of a single incident but was the culmination of a series of events that the staff found objectionable. Since Mr. Gray was the instigator of those events, one must, therefore, look at his culpability. Close examination suggests Mr. Gray's actions were motivated by appropriate concerns related to fiscal needs, quality of service, and staff development. Yet, despite Mr. Gray's seemingly positive motives and actions, he alienated his staff at every turn. If you agree that Mr. Gray's motives were not selfish and that his actions were reasonable, then you must look further to identify the true source(s) of Mr. Gray's culpability.

Most management authorities would attribute the blame for Mr. Gray's lack of success with his staff to his terse and insensitive method of communication. Given a situation in which there had been a greater exchange of information, concerns, and suggestions, it is quite possible the revolt would not have occurred.

Whether or not Mr. Gray has come to recognize his culpability in creating the problem, he nevertheless remains in a position in which he must make a decision. In fact, he must make his decision very soon. His task is not an easy one as this problem emphasizes the earlier contention that many administrative options involve subtle shades of gray rather than contrasting black and white. None of the alternatives carries a guarantee of satisfying all parties. When confronted with such a dilemma, one must strive to make the decision **most likely** to allay or resolve the problem.

Selected References

Ackoff, RL: The Art of Problem Solving. John Wiley, Chichester (Great Britain), 1978.

Culligan, MJ, and Deakins, CS, Young, AH: Back to Basics Management. Facts on File, New York, 1983.

Drucker, PF: Management—Tasks, Responsibilities, Practices. Harper & Row, New York, 1973.

Drucker, PF: Managing the Non-Profit Organization. Harper Collins, New York, 1990.

Eden, C, Jones, S, and Sims, D: Messing About in Problems: An Informal Structured Approach to Their Identification and Management. Pergamon Press, Oxford, 1983.

Hicks, MJ: Problem Solving in Business and Management. Chapman and Hall, London and New York, 1991.

Kepner, CH, and Tregoe, BB: The Rational Manager. McGraw-Hill, New York, 1965.

Kepner, CH, and Tregoe, BB: The New Rational Manager. Kepner-Tregoe, Inc., Princeton, 1981.

Kilmann, RH: Beyond the Quick Fix. Jossey-Bass, San Francisco, 1985.

Longest, BB Jr: Management Practices for the Health Professional. 3d edition, Reston Publishing, Reston, VA, 1984.

Nosse, LJ, and Frieberg, DG: Management Principles for Physical Therapists. Williams and Wilkins, Baltimore, 1992.

Phillips, SR, and Berquist, WH: Solutions—A Guide to Better Problem Solving. University Associates, San Diego, 1987.

Rakich, JS, Longest, BB Jr, and O'Donovan, TR: Managing Health Care Organizations. WB Saunders, Philadelphia, 1977.

Umiker, W: Management Skills for the New Health Care Supervisor. 2d edition, Aspen Publishers, Gaithersburg, MD, 1994.

Van Gundy, AB Jr: Techniques of Structured Problem Solving. 2d edition, Van Nostrand Reinhold, New York, 1988.

Index